With the compliments of
Farbwerke Hoechst AG

CANCER

A REVIEW OF INTERNATIONAL RESEARCH

CANCER

A REVIEW OF INTERNATIONAL RESEARCH

Ernst Bäumler

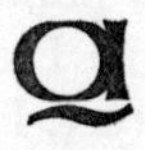

THE QUEEN ANNE PRESS LIMITED

English edition first published 1968

SBN 362 00039 5

First published in Germany by
Econ-Verlag GmbH, Dusseldorf and Vienna
This edition published by
The Queen Anne Press Limited,
49/50 Poland Street, London, W.1.,
and printed for them in Great Britain by
Tonbridge Printers Limited, Tonbridge, Kent

In memory
of
Irmgard Bäumler

CONTENTS

Acknowledgement of Illustrations

Rudi-Angenendt, Dortmund (3); Ballarin-Bild, Heidelberg (2); Chester Beatty Institute, London (2); German Cancer Research Centre, Heidelberg (2); dpa, Frankfurt-am-Main (1); Farbwerke Hoechst A.G. (12); National Institutes of Health, Bethesda, Maryland (3); Willi Pragher, Freiburg im Breisgau (1); Sloan Kettering Institute, New York (1); Veterans Administration Hospital, Bronx, New York (2).

PREFACE

For centuries a bitter duel has been fought, as mankind has endeavoured by every available means to ward off the most threatening enemy known to life: cancer. Victory over this ancient disease has often seemed almost within our grasp – the riddle of the malignant cell on the point of solution. But hope has always been followed by disillusionment and resignation, and confident forecasts by those involved in research have time and again proved false.

In our own time, despite tremendous efforts, cancer has still not been truly checked, let alone conquered. But how will the picture look in the future, in the next few decades? Where do we stand today in the battle against cancer? How do world-famous scientists regard the present situation, and the prospects in cancer research? Will the ultimate answer lie with surgery, with radiotherapy or chemo-therapy, or in the field of immunology?

The author of this book has sought the answers to these questions in interviews with many of the world's best-known authorities on cancer. In recent years he has had the opportunity of visiting most of the important cancer research institutes in Europe and the United States, and of learning the latest results of work going on there – not only on the latest methods of diagnosis and treatment of cancer, but also on the causes of the disease itself and possible means of preventing it.

The basic question of the cause and course of the malignant disease is one on which it can be claimed, without exaggeration, that a great many advances have been made in recent decades. To be sure, it is still very difficult to evaluate their significance in relation to the overall problem of cancer and its nature, and for this reason it cannot be prophesied in this book whether, or when, the ultimate riddle will be solved.

However, it is possible to define the spheres of research in which the most marked advances have been made. Only a few scientists still doubt that it is in two major areas of research – virology and immunology – that the most substantial successes will be achieved. Certainly, future success will depend upon developments in these two fields, and upon the conclusions drawn from countless new experiments.

No one today can venture a prophecy as to whether or when the doctor will have access to anti-cancer vaccines. The same is true of the end-products of many other lines of research discussed in this book. Molecular biology must certainly provide hard-core knowledge of the origin and cause of cancerous diseases. The American Nobel Laureate Linus Pauling once spoke of "sick (diseased) molecules". Cancer might just as well be defined as the "rogue" molecule. At all events, it is closely bound up with the nucleic acids, the chemical substances which make up those parts of the cell nucleus concerned with heredity. Increasing knowledge of the nucleic acid molecule clearly indicates the dramatic success achieved by biology and biochemistry in recent decades.

At the same time, nucleic acids have become the key compounds for study by cancer research workers, for there is little remaining doubt that all carcinogenic substances, be they chemicals or viruses, act on these acids to deform them and make them in a sense diseased. In this way, loss of the control of growth is caused – the one characteristic common in all cancer cells. Moreover, forms of cancer which appear without the discernible influence of external factors must have their origin in changes in the "molecule of life".

The advances made by research which are outlined in this book have been achieved painfully slowly, and the ultimate solution of the cancer problem will come too late for millions of people. Tragic though this may be, one cannot overlook the immensity of the tasks that face science: the process by which cells become malignant is one which lies beyond the normal laws of cell growth, and is obviously related closely to the mysteries of life itself. In a problem so immensely complex, we can hardly hope for accidental discoveries that will with one move tear the veil from the biological secrets so well concealed by nature.

For mankind there thus remains only a wearisome, step by step progress from discovery to discovery. This is precisely what happens in innumerable research laboratories today. Cancer research seems inseparably bound up with the growth of knowledge in general biology, biochemistry, embryology, genetics and many other disciplines.

However, it is today carried on all over the world – especially, as one would expect, in the United States – on a scale and with an intensity unprecedented in the history of human civilisation. This present account of these researches, therefore, although it must contain so many question marks and qualifications, cannot be regarded as in any way a pessimistic assessment. The French scholar and Nobel Laureate Charles Nicolle once considered that the cancer problem would never be solved, because it is beyond the comprehension of the human mind. Today, however, most research workers are convinced that Nicolle will ultimately be proved wrong.

Chapter 1

IT IS NEXT TO NOTHING

A simple chill develops with a multitude of symptoms. When heart disease threatens, the alarm is given in the form of increased blood pressure. Infectious diseases announce themselves with high temperatures and painful inflammations. Only one disease stalks its victim silently and without any symptom – as though the affected organism, confronted with the most dreadful illness of our time, has thoughtlessly abandoned its warning system. Theodor Storm, who died of gastric cancer, wrote:

> It is next to nothing
> A mere trifle, scarcely felt,
> And yet, a continual nuisance,
> Hard to explain in words
> If you wish to complain of it to others.
> You say to yourself, "It doesn't matter";
> But it still remains
> And the world becomes so strange
> That you lose all hope,
> And realise at last
> That you have indeed been stricken
> By the dread arrow of death!

Without any visible reason, the harmonious life of the cells is disturbed at a certain place in the organism. A single cell or a group of cells breaks away from the biological rhythm, withdraws from the infinite gradations of the regulatory system, and begins its own chaotic, independent life. No cell, no tissue, is secure from such a treacherous assault.

The reason for this revolt, this rejection of the organism's regulation, still baffles mankind today.

Many scientists believe that the initial phase of the disease begins with the first cancer cells. Everything depends on whether, and when, the first malignant cell will begin to divide and provide equally malignant descendents. This division need not occur immediately. Cancer cells do not always – as was thought for a long time – divide more readily than normal cells. There can be no other explanation of the 10–15 years that must usually elapse before the first cancer cells have multiplied to form a tumour.

Conceptions such as "initial phase" or "realisation phase", which refer especially to this lengthy development, are admittedly quite abstract; they are nothing more than an endeavour to divide the puzzling variety of cancerous processes into rough categories. In no other disease or group of diseases do we have to reckon with so many departures from the "rules". Cancer probably has a thousand faces!

Cells proliferate regardless of their neighbours

Before the cell was recognised as being the building block of all living things, many scholars believed that malignant tumours – or at least their first beginnings – came from outside the organism. Only since the middle of the last century has it been known that cancer cells only develop from other cells in the body. They are the progeny of normal cells, and are distinguished from these chiefly by a feature which is much more fundamental that a mere difference in rate of growth.

Normal cells are clearly able to recognise one another when, in the formation of tissue, they come together. When an individual cell makes contact with a neighbour, it ceases to divide and multiply. It respects, so to speak, its neighbour's territory.

The cancer cell is, by contrast, anarchistic. It divides regardless of the neighbouring cells, it penetrates foreign tissue. It establishes – by way of the blood vessels and the lymphatic system – colonies in widely separate parts of the body. It behaves in a hostile and aggressive manner.

All cancer cells have these characteristics, which stamp them as the most dangerous "law-breakers" in the biological community. "The cancer cell has its own laws and must obey them," said Charles Huggins, Director of the Ben-May Institute of Chicago University and 1966 Nobel Laureate for Medicine. The more rapidly the cancer cell divides, the more extensive is the "illegal" and malignant growth. And as the number of divisions increases, and as we move further and further away from the original, the cells themselves alter. They lose their original characteristics as the cells of a specific organ. Only remotely do they then resemble the cells from which they developed; they have become, above all, far more primitive – they have "undifferentiated" themselves. This is the reverse of "cell differentiation", a process which begins soon after the fertilisation of the female egg.

The development of a new individual from the first embryo cells proceeds by a process of continuous division. But this would produce no more than a formless heap of cells if the cells did not at the same time become differentiated, each to perform its special tasks. Some become blood cells, some go to form the liver, the brain and the other organs of the body. Nerve cells are the most specialised – the most highly differentiated – of all.

In the cancer cell, on the other hand, the "biological clock" is put back. The cell reverts to an unspecialised state, to a primitive form. In many cancer cells this happens to such a degree that pathologists can no longer determine exactly which organ they came from originally.

In the past it has been these advanced tumours whose cells have offered many cancer investigators their most important data for comparison with normal cells. Today, biochemical research concentrates on early cancer cells, which bear the greatest resemblance to healthy cells. This is especially true of cells from certain liver tumours. These are designated as "tumours of minimal deviation" – tumours whose constituents deviate only to a small degree from normal cells. This method offers the best hope of the eventual discovery of valid biochemical differences between healthy and malignant cells.

At the present time, however, even the most learned pathologist cannot always draw a clear line of distinction between the benign and the malignant. Asked what were the malignant characteristics of a cell, Dr Leslie Foulds of the Chester Beatty Institute, London, once replied: "Whether it kills the patient or not!"

The No-man's land between benign and malignant

The American cancer investigator, van Rensselaer Potter, Professor of Biochemistry at Madison University, Wisconsin, has studied extensively those tumours whose cells deviate least from healthy ones. He is one of the scientists who believe that the transition from the normal to the cancer cell is by way of an intermediate stage in which there are cells present which show the first signs of degeneracy but are still not definite cancer cells. They are defined as pre-cancerous, that is to say, cells in the preliminary stage of cancer.

When such cells which deviate from the normal – cells, so to speak, in the no-man's-land between benign and malignant – are found in vaginal scrapings, they present doctors with grave decisions. Ought one to operate at this stage? For these atypical cells are only in some cases cancerous. A normal cell can change into a potential cancer cell without any discernible cause. But this transformation can also be caused by an initiator – by a carcinogen, by a chemical cause of cancer, by ionising radiation and, at any rate in animals, by viruses.

Nevertheless, in most cases true cancer cells do not arise in this way. Only if further changes occur, or an associate cause comes to the aid of the primary carcinogen (a so-called catalyst in the form of a co-carcinogen) does the catastrophe then proceed further. The pre-cancerous cell changes into a *dependent* cancer cell. It is called *dependent* because it still obeys the laws of the cell community to some extent. If further factors act upon the dependent cancer cell, then it gives rise to the *autonomous* cancer cell. Only then has it irrevocably deserted its former community.

"The first step in the origin of cancer," said the East Berlin research worker U. Schneeweiss, "the cancerisation of the normal cell, is a cellular process. The second phase leads to the multiplication of the cancer cells, and to reciprocal interaction with the forces of the host."

Tragedy in three acts

Although scientists are by no means agreed that different phases of the development of cancer can be clearly distinguished, there is much experimental evidence that, in some forms of cancer, separate and definite events occur which ultimately result in the development of tumours. This is the belief of Dr. John Weisburger of the National Cancer Institute in the U.S.A.

The three stages from normal to cancer cells are called:

1. *Initiation.* The initial reaction between a carcinogen or the corresponding metabolic product with a certain constituent of the cell or tissue. In this way an abnormal and latent tumour cell, which cannot positively be differentiated under the microscope from a normal cell, is formed.
2. *Development.* The multiplication of these abnormal cells leads to visible tumour tissue. Presumably in this stage other environmental influences play a part, just as they were necessary for the initial phase.
3. *Progression.* Which includes all the fundamental changes in the nature of tumour cells.

Most important in this sequence is the first step – the initiation, because it marks the fundamental change from a normal to a tumour cell.

Probably this scheme – which applies especially to chemically-induced cancer – cannot be anything more than a provisional deduction based upon observations of experiments on animals. Most tumours develop by stages, and their behaviour and features differ widely from one another. Each new change makes the tumour cells more destructive, and destroys ever more markedly their capacity to perform normal functions. A cell need not, however, in all cases degenerate step by step. It can attain the stage of greatest malignancy at one leap.

The individual in whose body this has happened knows nothing of it. And that is the fateful thing: he does not notice, and believes himself to be perfectly healthy, although day by day cancer cells increase in a certain part of his body, until there is a tumour the size of a pinhead or a thimble. In the whole of this first stage of a cancerous disease, the cancer specialist rarely finds any clinically discernible symptoms.

Then this small cancer grows into a bigger tumour – though in this Stage II it is still restricted to its original site. This localised growth is still often overlooked, especially if it is hidden in an interior part of the body and does not yet exert pressure on vital or sensitive organs.

The third stage is the most dangerous

But finally the third stage begins: the cancer cells become more aggressive. They penetrate into the surrounding tissues, try to destroy them and appropriate all the growth and nutritional substances of the healthy tissue.

Only when this fatal stage has been reached, and when the cancer cells have begun their invasion of the healthy tissue, is the patient driven into the doctor's consulting room by pains and other symptoms that can no longer be ignored. Even then, some still delay. The ever increasing dread that it could be cancer paralyses their resolution and leads them deliberately to ignore the signs of disease. For the diagnosis of cancer is, for many people, equivalent to a sentence of death which will sooner or later be carried out with inexorable consistency.

What a tragic error this may be is proved by the record of cures (often unknown to the public) of cancer that has been diagnosed at an early stage. The further course of the disease, and prospects of cure, depend on early diagnosis, on the special character of the cancer cells and on the site of their growth. Several hundreds of different kinds of cancer are known, depending on the organ or tissue from which the malignant cells originate. It is this puzzling variety which has brought many scientists to regard the term cancer as no more than a general name for a whole group of diseases.

"Cancer is not a single disease but, fundamentally, a number of different diseases," said Dr. Charles Gordon Zubrod of the National Cancer Institute in the U.S.A. "That is the main conclusion of cancer research in recent years."

"This observation," Zubrod continued, "is admittedly in no way original. What is new is that today one seeks to attain control over 'cancer' by studying the individual diseases. It is also new that in at least two categories, the foundations of victory over these diseases have been laid."

How aggressive is a tumour?

Cancer is not *just* cancer, a lung tumour is not *just* a lung tumour and cancer of the stomach is not *just* cancer of the stomach. Every tumour has an unchangeable individuality; it can arise from quite different kinds of "cell lines". This variety of tumours is one of the main problems in treating the disease. "Different forms of malignant tumours show not only a different character, but also an individual *dynamic* in their development" said Professor Heinz Oeser, Head of the Radiological Institute of the Free University of Berlin. There are tumours which spread explosively and lead inevitably to death in the shortest time. But slow-growing malignant tumours are also known which exist for years or even decades. Between these two extremes there is a whole spectrum of development and growth forms. The "unlimited growth", which is one of the characteristics that differentiates tumour tissue from that of healthy organs, seems at first sight to be both unregulated and incalculable. For the last ten years doctors in the U.S.A. and many European countries have been at pains to define all observations quantitatively, so as to avoid concepts as generalised as "rapid" or "slow-growing". American research workers have established the thesis of "exponential" tumour growth, based on experimental studies of animal tumours.

If bacteria are transferred to cultures under favourable conditions of temperature, nutrient solutions, oxygen supply, etc., they divide with a definite rhythm. Because all the cells divide, their number is doubled in approximately constant periods of time. The total number thus increases in correspondence with a geometrical series of 1, 2, 4, 8 . . ., in mathematical formulation – an *exponential* function. Experimentally similar observations can also be made on tumour cells which have been maintained in culture. Here, too, an astonishing regularity can be observed. New cell generations always appear with twice the number of cells contained in the parent generation. But a tumour in the living organism develops in a manner that is fundamentally more complex than in the experiments just mentioned. This is only natural in view of the different nutritional structures, hormonal factors and defence systems of the body. "Nevertheless it seems justifiable," thinks Professor Oeser, "to take the theory of exponential growth as a basic working hypothesis for the investigation and interpretation of the development of cancer in man".

To measure the diameter and volume of a tumour exactly is possible only with superficial tumours of the skin, or in tumours (in man) that can be detected by X-rays. Experience in this field has therefore chiefly been obtained on such tumours. Röntgenograms allow exact measurements to be made of the size of tumours in cancer of the lung, and of secondary tumours in this organ. By further observation of their progress, the time it takes for the volume of the tumour to double can be estimated. This period is then defined as the "doubling time of the tumour", and constitutes a quantitative measure of "aggressiveness", and growth potential. This measure of time does not admittedly correspond directly to the multiplication time of the tumour cells, but is only a balance struck between all the processes of cell-renewal and cell-death in the tumour. Much still depends upon the variable vitaility and division-rate of the cells.

Surprising results have come from the working hypothesis of exponential growth. The whole developmental period of a tumour is considered from the initial stages with a few cells to a tumour with many millions of cells. Thirty to thirty-five cell-generations are necessary before a clinically demonstrable tumour develops from the first groups. At this moment the growth of the cancer cells seems to proceed like an avalanche, though the long duration of this process still remains largely hidden. This temporal course has been compared to an iceberg, the greater part of which remains invisible. Three-quarters of the life span of a cancer has been completed before clinical signs and discomforts appear, and before it can be diagnosed even by the best methods of investigation.

Remarkable as are the advances made in recent years in surgical, radiological and chemotherapeutic treatment, there are still many kinds of cancer which, in these later stages, can only be temporarily checked.

As Oeser explained: "the quantitative considerations of cancer growth and the temporal dynamic make it possible to explain many hitherto obscure phenomena, and many failures despite the best possible treatment. It is to be hoped that improved knowledge of the developmental phases of cancer will bring experience to enable the doctor to help his patient more speedily and effectively."

What, therefore, is to be done? Naturally, new and better chemical weapons against cancer are being sought. Nevertheless it is just as important to investigate all the methods by which cancer can be diagnosed and treated at an earlier stage. The ideal would naturally be a general cancer test, perhaps a blood examination, which would give clear information as to whether a person harbours cancer cells or not.

At the present time such a biological test – like the Wassermann reaction in syphilis – is nowhere in sight. In a blood test one of the signs of cancer is an increased sedimentation rate of the red blood corpuscles. But this phenomenon also occurs in a fairly large number of other diseases. Although it appears doubtful whether cancer cells leave behind "finger-prints", many American cancer research institutes are working with great intensity on a biochemical cancer test. This starts from the – admittedly unproven – theory that, in cancer patients, biochemical changes should be discernible long before the first demonstrable symptoms appear. In these investigations blood has been taken annually from a large circle of people. The blood plasma is carefully stored. If somebody in this group subsequently develops cancer, or another disease, his blood plasma can be compared with that from the period when no signs of disease were yet discernible. Whether in this way wide and generally valid differences become evident – long before the cancer would be diagnosed by methods in use today – it will only be possible to say after a number of years. In any case this is a fascinating experiment which has become possible only since the discovery how to preserve biological material at extremely low temperatures. By means of liquid nitrogen, it is now possible to reduce blood plasma to minus 130 degrees to 196 degrees C; at this point the molecular biological activity falls to zero and the enzymes and other important constituents of the cell can be preserved intact.

Seven signals of alarm . . .

At present, early diagnosis must depend on very imprecise symptoms. The initial symptoms to which each individual should pay attention have been summarised by the American Cancer Society under seven headings.

1. Unusual haemorrhages or secretions.
2. A nodule or thickening in the breast or elsewhere.
3. A wound or scar that will not heal.
4. Changes in the alimentary canal or bladder region.
5. Persistent hoarseness or cough.
6. Digestive troubles or difficulty in swallowing.
7. Marked changes in a wart or birth mark (naevus).

If one of these alarm signals lasts longer than two weeks, see your doctor: it may indicate cancer. Though this list may seem to be trivial, life or death may depend on following its warnings.

The American Cancer Society continually hammers away at the American people with striking statistics: every second sufferer from cancer can today be saved, if the diagnosis is made in time and the treatment can begin early enough. There are about 1.2 million people living now in the United States who have been cured of cancer or, to put it more accurately, who are without any signs of cancer 5 years after the end of treatment.

A unique Institution...

The American Cancer Society was founded in 1913. As a purely private association it has today more than 2 million subscribing and active members. Its annual budget, based entirely upon gifts, finances research programmes, cancer clinics, the collection of statistics and educational campaigns. In 1964 this institution, the only one of its kind in the world, supported 478 research projects in 173 American institutes. The scope of these research efforts included all aspects of the cancer problem: questions of cell life, growth and ageing, cell diseases and the process of their death. "Since all this," says a publication of the Society, "has to do with the cancer problem, either directly or indirectly."

Special research problems are: what is a virus? How does a cell convey its hereditary structure to its descendants? Why are some cells susceptible to cancer while others are not? How do hormones intervene in the growth process? Why do cells become old and why do they die? How do the chemical control reactions of the cell work? How is it that cancer cells come to lie in ambush in the human body, apparently quiescent for years, before they suddenly begin to attack a vital organ?

Admittedly this extensive research programme, which the Society first began in 1945, still contains many gaps. For example, only 23 research workers received support in the field of virology, although this is one of the most promising and important areas of study. Only one scientist in this programme is working on skin cancer, a form of cancer from which about 68,000 people in America suffered in 1963 alone. Only five of the scientists supported by the Society worked on cancer of the intestine, a disease to which 46,000 Americans annually fall victims.

These examples do not justify the complacent thinking of many European States and Health Ministers. The alleged fact that the Americans have fought on the cancer front ostensibly without financial limit, and have been able to undertake any research project that promises results without regard to the cost, is, for the government authorities of other countries, sufficient excuse for a totally inadequate investigation of cancer, towards which the efforts of all civilised countries should be devoted. Professor Hans

Erhard Bock, President of the German Cancer Society, is very critical in this connection of West Germany, where only £450,000 is available each year for cancer research "We have far too little money, and must consider how vital investigations into the chemotherapy of cancer can be financed in the future," complained Bock in 1966 to the Munich Cancer Congress.

The situation in Great Britain

In England, on the other hand, about 6 times the sum named by Bock for the Federal Republic of Germany is allocated for cancer research. Professor Sir Alexander Haddow, Director of the Chester Beatty Institute, estimated the annual cost to his country of this work at about £3,500,000. About half of this, so Haddow believes, comes from private sources, whilst the state contributes the other 50 per cent.

Thus in London an annual collection is organised, the proceeds of which are available alternately to the two big organisations specifically engaged in the battle against cancer: the British Empire Cancer Campaign for Research and the Imperial Cancer Research Fund. The former supports research in hospitals and institutes of the country. The latter, on the other hand, maintains its own research centre, the scientific staff of which co-operate with doctors and surgeons in other clinics. Sometimes working groups are also sent overseas, for example, to investigate epidemic lymphoma in Africa. The scientific work of the centre is concentrated on human cancer, especially on leukaemia, cancer of the breast and prostate, and on viruses causing cancer.

In 1965 the ICRF provided a staff of more than 300 scientists and technicians and worked with a budget of £1,806,000. This sum came from private sources without any State support. The biggest contributions were bequests to the extent of £914,000. Membership contributions, donations and fund-raising activities brought in £683,000, whilst the remainder of the income came from interest and dividends.

In the Federal Republic of Germany there is no organisation comparable to this, which collects information on cancer on such a broad basis and at the same time allocates large sums for cancer research. The study of cancer in the Federal Republic lies chiefly in the hands of regional authorities, by far the most active of which is the North Rhineland Westphalian Society for Combating Cancerous Diseases.

In contrast to the American Cancer Society, this is not an organisation with millions of helpers and benefactors, but a small group of twenty-two specialists, its annual budget being about £200,000 granted by the State Parliament in Düsseldorf from public funds. More extensive organisations, thinks their Chairman, Professor Dr. Wilhelm Flaskamp, "often suffer from too large a membership which hinders the work". One of the most important tasks, in his opinion, is the explanation of the facts to a wide population. The laity should "be told of the most important symptoms of the disease and encouraged to acquire self knowledge and to study precautionary measures". At the same time, fear of the disease should be removed by information about successful cures. Flaskamp repeatedly emphasises that "cancer is curable". But only if it is treated in time.

To such instruction of the laity the Society devotes every effort, using lectures, pamphlets, books, films and publications in the Press. "We have even organised theatrical performances," Flaskamp recollects. Medical education is allied to these endeavours. It was especially important at the time when the Society was formed, in 1950, when following the war, there was a lack of trained doctors, of hospitals, of laboratories, and even of books and other facilities.

Therefore the Society organised numerous lectures and special courses, founded a free information service, which reported on the new results of research, and set up a central library, which today contains more than 15,000 volumes of international cancer literature.

This work is still carried on, and now Professor Flaskamp insists that "war damage" has been completely overcome. "In treatment we have today reached an international standard and have no need to fear any comparison." The Society also established local regional centres. In these consulting places women can be examined, free of charge, for cancer. In 186 such centres between 1952 and 1965, a total of 504,372 women were examined. In 7,115, or 1.41 per cent, hitherto undiagnosed cancer was found.

Such diagnoses are in every case inseparably linked with cytological investigations by the Pap smear method, and for this reason the Society founded 10 cytological centres. "We have so far published the results of the examinations of 683,587 patients in our 10 centres," Professor Flaskamp reports. "We have thus realised the most extensive programme of early diagnosis known to world literature."

An important part of the work of these centres is also the training of doctors in cytological methods. "The central laboratory of Professor H. K. Zinser in Cologne is one of the largest and best known in the world, and in 1965 alone a total of 328 European and overseas doctors received instruction there.'

Whilst the cytological centres are considered to be permanent organisations, the Society is considering the reduction of the number of its clinics, since the work they do can now be undertaken to an increasing degree by individual gynaecologists.

Until 1965 there was in the Federal Republic no central research centre comparable to the large institutes in the U.S.A. or Great Britain. First to be built was the German cancer research centre in Heidelberg, organised by a group of the leading German cancer investigators (the so-called Hinterzartener Kreis), the foundation stones of which were laid in November 1964.

When the institute is complete, about 200 scientists will work in it. Since the autumn of 1966 it has possessed a research reactor for the production of short-life radioactive substances. Isotope laboratories, an electronic computer in which all the knowledge about cancer can be stored, and a fully air-conditioned and sterile unit for 10,000 experimental animals are to be added.

S.O.S. from a cancer investigator

Professor Karl Heinrich Bauer, doyen of German cancer investigators and Administrator of the Heidelberg research centre, hopes that the Federal Republic will through this regain international status. To be sure, this can only happen if the Federal Government undertakes more energetic promotion of the cause of cancer research, which has been hitherto somewhat neglected. The emergency call, which Professor Hans Lettré, Director of the Institute of Experimental Cancer Research in the University of Heidelberg and one of the most renowned investigators of cancer, put out in August, 1965, on German television, could also come from many other research centres with limited financial resources. "Our request to the public and state authorities, is that sufficient money be placed at our disposal to permit us to concentrate our labours exclusively on our special tasks. It is not right that we have to devote 80 per cent of our working time to the provision of money for the work."

Though the Heidelberg cancer research centre is especially concerned with scientific fundamentals, another institution devotes itself particularly to case studies. In Essen, this is a clinical research Institute under the direction of Professor Dr. Carl Gottfried Schmidt of Munster, one of the best known German experts in cytostatics.

The plan for this clinic, which is managed by the Chair of Internal Medicine of the Essen clinic of the University of Munster, was prepared by the North Rhineland Westphalian Society for Combating Cancerous Diseases. The financial support of £3,500,000 was provided by the central Government and the City of Essen.

Of some 200 beds planned, two thirds should serve the oncological division and the other third the projected radiological clinic. The clinical sections were completed and began work in 1967.

The completion of a supplementary laboratory is provided for in 3 year's time. In addition to standard equipment, this building will contain "hot" laboratories and animal houses, in which work can be done with radioactive material. Moreover, for the first time in the Federal Republic, there will be completely sterile sick rooms for special treatments, such as chorionepitheliomas and bone marrow transplantations.

Medical examinations on collective farms

In the Soviet Union there are several central institutes in which cancer research is carried out on a broad basis. Special importance is also ascribed to mass campaigns for the early diagnosis of cancer. "All males over 35 and all women over 30 must be examined at least once a year," says Professor A. N. Novikov, Director of the Alexander Herzen Institute for oncology in Moscow. "In 1963 20 million people were examined in the Soviet Union and this mass undertaking, begun in 1948, is to be further intensified."

Such measures are carried out at a cost and with an intensity which are possible only in a totalitarian state. Regular and systematic examinations are carried out at all factories, collective farms and offices. Even residential blocks have their own consulting room, in which the tenants can and must accept medical advice, especially regarding symptoms of cancer. Whoever does not make use of this facility receives a friendly but firm letter which explains that attending lectures on the early diagnosis of cancer is in his own specific interest. But the State is not satisfied even with that. It obliges every doctor, whether a practitioner, specialist or even a dentist, to report immediately any suspicion of cancer.

If such a suspicion is verified by more accurate investigation, the patient is immediately treated in a special clinic, health centre, military clinic, or in the State cancer institute. Naturally, cancer-medicine in the Soviet Union is organised extremely strictly and bureaucratically. At its head is the oncological division of the Health Ministry. Subordinate to this are the distinguished Alexander Herzen Institute and the Institute for Experimental and Clinical Oncology, which belongs to the Academy of Medical Sciences. All the leading cancer specialists of the Soviet Union co-operate with this oncological Institute.

The specialists continuously check on the ability of their colleagues working in the health centres. If any short-comings are discovered, the doctor concerned must take a special course of instruction. 50,000 doctors attend such courses annually.

The need for early diagnosis

Soviet scientists also lay special emphasis on methods for the early diagnosis of cancer. In this they start from the assumption that there is a precancerous stage, in which the molecular weight of the blood differs from that of healthy people. Since 1960 intensive work has been going on in the Soviet Union on a method for showing the structure of the blood graphically.

In the Soviet Union it is believed that before cancer appears in a certain spot, changes in the whole organism must occur. The Russian cancer investigator Professor L. A. Shabad, maintains that "many pathological processes and tissue changes initially lay the foundations for a cancer. If we do not think from the first of the possibility of a cancerous disease, we miss the right moment for early diagnosis and early treatment. In my opinion, treatment of the early stage is the best way to cure cancer."

But in spite of all early diagnosis cancer still takes a high toll: in 1963 about 280,000 people died of it in the U.S.A. – 800 a day, or one every 2 minutes. In the Federal Republic of Germany the annual death rate from cancer amounts to 120,000, so that the proportion of the total population is even higher than it is in the U.S.A. Europe has, moreover, the highest cancer mortality in the whole world. Whilst, for example, for every 100,000 of the population, the average number of annual cancer deaths, in recent years, was 330 in West Berlin, 256 in Austria and 185 in Czechoslovakia, there were in the U.S.A. only 149, in Canada only 129, and in Japan, which has the highest death rate from cancer in the Far East, only 102. Altogether the World Health Organisation estimated that in 1964, throughout the world, there were at least 5 million sufferers, from cancer.

According to a publication of the American Cancer Society, the frequency of different kinds of cancer in males and females is entirely different. 29 per cent of cancer occurring in men are cancers of the digestive system. About 18 per cent are cancers of the respiratory system, trachea, bronchi and lungs. About 14 per cent suffer from genital and skin cancer, about 8 per cent from leukaemia and lymphoma, 6 per cent from tumours of the urinary tract, 4 per cent have cancer of the buccal cavity. The remaining 7 per cent show various less common kinds of cancer.

In women sufferers, on the other hand, cancer of the breast takes first place with 25 per cent, followed by genital cancer and cancer of the digestive tract, 23 per cent each. 10 per cent of women suffer from skin cancer, 5 per cent from leukaemia and lymphoma taken together, and only 3 per cent each from cancer of the urinary tract and – most surprisingly – from cancer of the respiratory organs. In women cancer of the buccal cavity plays a still smaller part, being only 1 per cent. The sad remainder of 7 per cent corresponds with the findings in men.

Lung cancer has progressively become one of the chief causes of death in males. About 5 times as many males as females suffer from it – most of them between the ages of 50 and 70 years. In the Federal Republic of Germany the marked increase of lung cancer has led to a higher cancer death-rate in men than in women. Out of 1,000 men 206 died of cancer of the lung, trachea and bronchi, but only 35 women. The first symptom of lung cancer is persistent cough and mucous expectoration. The sputum may be stained with blood. In the later stages the growing tumour destroys the bronchi.

Endoscopy helps to diagnose tumours

The diagnosis of lung tumours still causes trouble for clinicians. Radioscopy, investigations of the sputum and of cells obtained from the bronchi, and the technique of bronchoscopy, are the chief methods of investigation. The bronchoscope is an instrument with an inbuilt illuminating system, with which specific areas of the lungs can be accurately inspected.

There is a whole arsenal of these optical tubes, ranging from the simple short tube, the rectoscope, for investigating the rectum, to a yard-long, semi-rigid system of lenses, prisms and lights, for the investigation of the interior of the stomach (the gastroscope). Endoscopy, in fact, is an important aid to the early diagnosis of cancer.

In the past, when lung cancer was suspected, an extensive operation of exploratory thoracotomy was often necessary. This involved dividing the ribs and opening the thorax. Mediastinoscopy, a procedure developed by Swedish surgeons, has recently provided greatly improved chances of diagnosis and in many cases makes exploratory thoracotomy unnecessary. For mediastinoscopy an incision must first be made into the jugular fossa on the anterior aspect of the neck, and the trachea must be exposed. A way is then cleared through which the mediastinoscope can be introduced. The instrument makes it possible to look at the trachea, the aorta and the other large vessels in the mid-thoracic region and the surrounding lymphatic glands. This relatively trifling incision, following which the patient can go home after a day in hospital, helps in most cases to achieve a sound diagnosis.

If a lung carcinoma is diagnosed in time, the most effective treatment is pneumectomy, in which the diseased lobe of the lung is removed along with the regional lymphatic glands. Unfortunately more than 70 per cent of all lung tumours are only detected when it is too late for the surgeon, because the first secondary tumours have already settled in other parts of the body. X-ray treatment and chemotherapy, especially with nitrogen-mustard compounds, may even in these cases prolong life and alleviate the lot of the patient.

Is the cigarette entirely to blame?

In no other field of cancerous disease have investigators and clinicians sought so eagerly to explain the cause as in cancer of the lung. Researches on it are legion. At the end of 1964 an American Research Commission announced that it had worked for a year through a mountain of such material from all over the world. "There is a causal relationship between cigarette smoking and lung cancer." This was the so-called "Terry Report". It was not news for most investigators of cancer. The distinguished American cancer investigator Professor Ernest L. Wynder, for example, of the New York Sloan-Kettering Institute, said, "For me a discussion on the carcinogenic effect of the cigarette is as superfluous as a debate on the question of whether the earth may be flat!"

Wynder reported that in New York only about one case of lung cancer is annually observed in non-smokers. The risk run by heavy smokers of developing cancer of the lung is about 40 times greater than it is among non-smokers. Wynder is passionate and embittered when he speaks of this problem and of the "ostrich attitude of many cigarette smokers".

Nature has, in the course of millions of years, developed a defence system which is situated in the nose and protects the body from foreign substances. She could surely not foresee that in the 20th century both the mouth and throat would suddenly be invaded by such foreign bodies. The smoke of every cigarette contains 60–70 million particles. Whether cigarette smoking is therefore the only cause of bronchial cancer or whether other causes also exist is for many cancer investigators a question of purely secondary significance.

What part does alcohol play?

Wynder has, however, declared war not only on the cigarette but also on alcohol. He commented ironically at the 14th Congress for Medical Education in Berlin: "As I began to preach that the cigarette is to blame for lung cancer, I lost some of my friends. As I warned that whisky drinking can cause cancer of the mouth and oesophagus, I lost still more, and since I told people that nuns do not develop cancer of the uterus, I have been completely isolated."

In New York clinics half of all the patients with buccal and oesophageal cancer are alcoholics. The New York Academy of Sciences published in this connection the results of investigations which, in fact, supply no conclusive proof of a relationship between the consumption of alcohol and cancer, but nevertheless deserve consideration.

In these investigations the seeds of edible onions were germinated on filter paper. Part of this filter paper was soaked in pure water, but the other part in solutions whose defects were to be investigated. When the roots of the unions were ½ to 1 cm long, the seeds were examined to discover whether cell changes could be observed in them, similar to those found after exposure to radiation. Surprisingly, such changes were found in onion seeds whose "filter paper cultivation" had been treated with some solutions. After germination of the onions in a 1 per cent solution of ethyl alcohol, the cell changes corresponded to a daily radiation dose of 40 Röntgens. Caffeine in the concentration of a normal cup of coffee was equal to a daily radiation dose of 30–50 Röntgens. When one remembers that the American Atomic Energy Commission has established a weekly dose of only 0.1 Röntgen as the highest limit of safety for employees exposed to radiation, then these results merit attention.

Perhaps the explanation of the fact that alcoholics are more often affected by cancer of the mouth and oesophagus than other people is concealed in these results.

The campaign against cigarettes and alcohol can be carried on at present only with statistical evidence. A direct biological demonstration is still lacking. It will presumably be lacking as long as cancer remains un-identified in biochemical detail inside the cell.

In lung cancer other factors than cigarettes are also involved. The air in large towns has a high concentration of carcinogens. The effect of combustion gases from households and industry, the exhaust gases of automobiles and even the street dust in which Joachim Borneff, Professor of Hygiene at Mainz, has found carcinogenic particles – all contribute some effect.

Smoking has scarcely been affected by the warnings from cancer research workers and the Terry Report. Thus the consumption of cigarettes in the Federal Republic of Germany, which was about ninety thousand million in 1964, increased to ninety-five thousand million in 1965. Even the members of the Terry Commission have not been induced to give up smoking after their report!

In cancer of the stomach – or cancer of the digestive organs in general – there is no conclusive proof that substances in human food are responsible, but the number of scientists who ascribe a secondary causatory role to certain kinds of food and eating habits is on the increase.

Carcinoma of the stomach is one of the most dangerous forms of cancer. The only therapy promising results must in most cases be the radical removal of the whole stomach, or at least the greater part of it – together with the regional lymph glands. In operable cases only about 30 per cent of patients can be saved in this way. This percentage is comparatively low, because in most cases cancer of the stomach is not discovered in time. The first symptoms are usualy quite vague and only seldom lead the person affected by them to the doctor: ill-health, difficulty in swallowing, nausea, exhaustion and unexplained aversion to meaty foods. Later, marked loss of weight an anaemia occur as accompanying symptoms.

Early X-ray examinations, constant controls of weight, stool examination for blood, blood tests and blood albumin examinations, as well as cytological investigations, chemical analyses of the gastric juice and gastroscopy, all belong to today's diagnostic vocabulary which is still imperfect.

In spite of all this, clinicians have often found it difficult to distinguish between chronic gastric ulcer and a malignant tumour. It may happen that a carcinoma is favourably influenced for a time by the treatment of an ulcer. Many doctors take the precaution of regarding a gastric ulcer in older men which does not readily heal as being "precancerous" and eventually malignant. A conclusive diagnosis can often only be made by surgical examination of the interior of the stomach.

Gastric cancer on the retreat

Although the picture presented by gastric cancer is so unsatisfactory and although this type of cancer has such a poor prognosis – the future outlook is more hopeful. In many countries gastric cancer is on the retreat to an astonishing degree. Experts are not altogether agreed about the reason for this, but investigators who believe that cancer is due to external causes ascribe it, especially in America, to improved nutritional conditions and the greater consumption of fresh fruit and vegetables. It may be no accident that cancer is still very common wherever foods poor in vitamins predominate.

If this explanation is correct, gastric cancer must decline still further in coming years. Many substances have already been banned from human food, including certain preservatives which one may at least accept as under suspicion of causing cancer. This is true, for instance, of the pigment butter-yellow, which seems to have played a certain part not only in cancer of the liver but also in cancer of the stomach, though admittedly its carcinogenicity has only been established in experiments on animals.

Dr. Papanicolaou helps women

Abdominal cancer in women is today usually diagnosed quite early and cured – a fact which is not true of cancer of the lung and stomach. The procedure used is as simple as it is effective, and has saved innumerable women from death. In America it is popularly known as the 'Pap smear', after the name of its discoverer Dr. George N. Papanicolaou of the New York Hospital Cornell Medical Center.

Dr. "Pap", as his students call him, based the development of his test on the fact that cells are naturally shed by all tissues in the same way that the skin peels off after a sunburn. Thus, in the female vagina, cells from the uterus are found. These cells mostly lie in a certain amount of fluid, but if they are scraped off and fixed, they can be examined under the microscope and the cytologist can easily differentiate the atypical, i.e. diseased, cells from the healthy ones.

By this method cancer is diagnosed months or years before the first symptoms normally appear. By far the commonest and most dangerous cancer of the uterus, cancer of the cervix uteri, can nowadays be diagnosed by this method, which is used in almost every large clinic, and treated before it becomes dangerous.

This cancer of the uterus, which usually grows very slowly, over a period of 5–10 years, is often cured in time, and the chances of cure have increased to a gratifying degree. On an average the prospects of cure after early diagnosis vary between 75 per cent and 100 per cent – a quota of results that is unique in the treatment of cancer. With late diagnosis, this figure, of course, falls rapidly. It is, in most German clinics, about 50 per cent.

Breast Cancer is also cured

The commonest form of cancer in women – cancer of the breast – has also lost some of its terrors. Many women nowadays take heed of suspicious changes in the breast. There are nowadays better clinical methods of investigation, such as mammography and taking samples of the soft tissue of the affected mammary glands. Thus the prospects of cure have been greatly improved. Unfortunately, benign and malignant tumours cannot be clearly differentiated by mammography and therefore a biopsy is often essential, as it is in other forms of cancer. A small piece of tissue is removed from the growth suspected to be cancer and this is examined for malignancy by pathologists. Usually this is done immediately after the surgeon has exposed the affected part of the breast. While the patient is still on the operating table under the anaesthetic, a quick section – a section of the diseased tissue as thin as a film – is examined under the microscope. The decision as to whether it is benign or malignant is made in 10–12 minutes.

If it is found to be malignant the whole breast gland, together with the cancerous nodule, is removed. Naturally the patient has been asked beforehand whether this may be done, provided that the tumour proves to be malignant. But in every case valuable time is saved by this procedure, as is double anaesthesia and a second operation. The tumour is removed in this operation with the electric knife, the diathermy knife. The risk that malignant cells may be carried by the blood to other parts of the body is reduced in this way to a minimum, and the lymphatic glands can also be closed immediately.

Doctors urgently recommend that women should have their breasts examined several times a year. But as this is difficult to achieve many American doctors have changed to advising women how to carry out self-examination. The American Cancer Society has produced publications and films about this, to familiarise women with the technique.

The most important thing here, as it is in all other forms of cancer, is that the treatment must begin before secondary tumours, metastases, have been sown in other parts of the body, often far away from the primary tumour.

A million cells as a start

Such dangerous secondary tumours presumably grow in four stages, as Professor Dietrich Schmähl, Director of the Institute for Experimental Tumour Production and Treatment in the German cancer research centre at Heidelberg, suggested in February, 1966, at the German Cancer Congress in Munich.

First some single cells separate from the primary tumour. These are washed away by the blood and lymph. Cancer cells may be detached from the primary tumour by mechanical means, for example during operations or under pressure, or by chemical factors. It is believed that a lack of calcium favours their detachment because cells are held together by calcium, though surprisingly, small tumours often disseminate cells much earlier than large ones. The reason for this is as yet unknown.

Once cancer cells have been shed into the blood, the next stage in the establishment of metastases follows – the floating cells settle in a certain part of the body. For this to happen, however, the number of cells detached must be at least a million. Smaller numbers of cells usually die slowly in the blood or lymph.

This dissemination of cancer cells is followed by the development of secondary tumours. American investigators have been able to establish that substances which inhibit the coagulation of the blood apparently also hinder the formation of secondary tumours. These observations, however, have so far been made only in experiments on animals. It does not follow that they correspond to the conditions in man. But this could open up a hopeful line of research.

Radio isotopes as "tracers"

Important advances in the early diagnosis of cancer have been made with the aid of radio isotopes. These are transformations of elements, which are chemically exactly the same, but whose atomic nuclei break down and, in the process, emit radiation.

Such isotopes are today used as "tracers" in the diagnosis of cancer. This method provides various possibilities. On the one hand, the radio-active element, either in its pure form or in combination with a "carrier" which is stored preferentially by the cancer cells, is introduced into the tumour. Among such substances is phosphorus, and its isotope is used in successful diagnosis of tumours of the eyes and brain. If the radioactive atoms have accumulated in the malignant tissue, they can be "located" by radiation detectors and the tumour stands out against its healthy environment as a "hot nodule".

In this way tumours about 3 cm in diameter and with a volume of about 14 cc can be detected. Professor Hans Oeser, Director of the Radiological Institute of the Free University in Berlin, says that "the earlier a tumour lying deep in the body is detected, the greater must be the difference in activity between the tumour region and its environment".

The situation is especially favourable in many tumours of the thyroid gland. The healthy thyroid normally stores up iodine. Malignant cells of the thyroid tissue, also, often retain the ability to do this. If the patient is given a radioactive "iodine cocktail" to drink, the radio-detector makes it possible to detect not only the gland tumour, but sometimes also metastases formed from the malignant tissue in other parts of the body.

In contrast to the concentration of isotopes in the tumour, the opposite can also occur, so that the cancerous tissue remains "cold", whilst the surrounding healthy tissue absorbs the radioactive substance. The detection of such "cold nodules", Oeser emphasizes, is certainly more difficult than the search for "hot" areas. However, diagnostic results are possible in this way also, especially the early diagnosis of metastases in the liver.

A third method has only recently been developed by Dr. Helmut Ernst of the Radiology Clinic in the Free University of Berlin – this method is called Zintigraphy of the lung. It uses large albumen molecules containing radioactive iodine 131. If the blood supply of the lung tissue, especially in the bronchi and root of the lung, is affected by tumours, then the radioactive substance becomes dammed up there and the area affected can be, so to speak, illuminated from within.

Perhaps, one day, biochemists will succeed in developing a general cancer test. At the moment the diagnosis of tumours with the aid of radionucleides is decidedly preferable. A blood test would only show that cancer cells were present in the organism. Their whereabouts could not be detected. Radionucleides, on the other hand, show exactly where the tumour is hidden.

In addition to radionucleides, the X-ray screen has an important place in early diagnosis. This holds good for the simple X-ray picture and also for photographs, in which tumours can be identified with the aid of contrast media. Cancers of the bladder, ureter, pelvis or the kidney, tumours of the spinal cord and brain, are often detected by this method, though they must have reached a certain size before they can be made visible.

The terminology of malignancy

Malignancy also has its own terminology: carcinoma are defined as malignant tumours starting from the skin or mucous membranes such as those of the breast, prostate, thyroid gland or uterus. Sarcoma on the other hand are tumours of the connective or supporting tissues, the muscles, bones or nerves. Terms such as lung tumours, brain tumour, or skin cancer are always inclusive expressions. Among malignant brain tumours alone there are 3 chief types: tumours in the brain tissue itself (gliomas), medulloblastomas and glioblastomas. Prospects of cure are at their best in the case of gliomas. If treatment is given in time, the patient may, according to the site of the tumours and their histological constitution, live for many years without symptoms or trouble.

The prognosis of the various kinds of skin cancer is quite different. In the melanoblastomas the prospects of cure are about 50 per cent. But in the other forms (spinaliomas) it can be increased to almost 100 per cent.

Revolt among the leucocytes

In contrast to all these solid tumours, leukaemia, especially feared in children, plays a special rôle in the kaleidoscope of cancer. Although it has been a clear clinical concept for more than a hundred years, there was for a long time no agreement as to whether it fitted, as a disease of the haemopoietic organs, into the category of cancer. After the Second World War, however, leukaemia was definitely included by the World Health Organisation (WHO) under the heading of cancer in the list of causes of death.

The course and prospects of cure of this disease are just as diverse as are the methods of treatment. First it must be decided whether it is a case of lymphocytic leukaemia or of the so-called granulocytic leukaemia. The lymphocytic form affects the white blood cells formed in the lymph nodes, which are about the size of a lentil or a hazel nut and situated at intervals along the lymphatic vessels. Granulocytic, or as it is also called myeloid leukaemia, is caused by over-production of granulocytes, which are white cells produced by the bone marrow, the nuclei of which contain granular structures.

There are acute and chronic variants of both of these forms of leukaemia. In acute leukaemia the white blood corpuscles multiply themselves to an excessive extent. They become larger than normal, but are immature and incapable of functioning as healthy white cells. In a healthy person there are normally 5,000–10,000 cells of this kind per cubic millimetre. The same amount of blood in a patient suffering from leukaemia contains up to 500,000 of them.

The more these immature leucocytes inundate the blood, the more they hinder the formation of normal white and red corpuscles. This often results in anaemia, owing to a deficit of red blood cells. If the number of white cells is again reduced, susceptibility to infection increases, because the immature leucocytes cannot carry out their defensive rôle against invading micro-organisms. At the same time the number of blood platelets is markedly reduced in leukaemic patients. Because these thrombocytes play an important part in the coagulation of the blood, leukaemia is often accompanied by haemorrhages.

In chronic leukaemia the white blood cells are not so immature as they are in the acute form, and can combat bacteria to a certain degree.

Although infections and haemorrhages are only concomitant symptoms of leukaemia, they cause about 80 per cent of the severe complications or fatal cases of the disease. Other symptoms of leukaemia are fever, pains in the limbs and joints, enlargements of the lymph nodes and of the spleen and liver.

The first signs: abnormal cells in the blood

Before these symptoms appear, leukaemia is usually detected in its early stages by routine blood tests. First symptoms of the disease include abnormal weakness, striking pallor of the face, anaemia and haemorrhages. The number of leucocytes may at this stage already have increased, but may also still be normal. Abnormal cells in the blood or bone marrow usually provide clues for the first diagnosis.

What induces this hypertrophy of the bone marrow and lymphatic tissue, and their mass production of white cells?

The ultimate cause of it in leukaemia is still unknown, as it is in other forms of cancer. But ionising rays must certainly be held at least jointly responsible, just as are certain chemicals. Thus the incidence of leukaemia among the survivors of the Hiroshima atom bomb explosion is 20–30 times higher than normal. Patients who are irradiated for diagnostic or therapeutic purposes – and medical radiologists – develop leukaemia more often than other people. On the other hand ionising rays are not the only causes of leukaemia. Many people suffering from it have never been subjected to such rays.

It is easier to explain leukaemia in the children of women who have undergone radiological study or treatment during pregnancy. In suckling children the disease is usually combined with other congenital conditions, such as mongolism or bone-marrow defects. One belief, among others, is that influences and disturbances in the early weeks of pregnancy may cause leukaemia in the unborn child.

One chromosome too many

In many animals there is no doubt that hereditary influences play a direct part in leukaemia, but there is no proof that this is the case in humans. However, there is much to be said for the idea that leukaemia is often associated with abnormalities in the hereditary structure. A definite relationship between mongolism and leukaemia has certainly become evident. It has been shown recently that the inborn mental impairment depends on a "defect in the distribution of the chromosomes in the formation of the egg cells". A normal person contains about 20 thousand million body cells. In each nucleus of this astronomical number of cells there are 46 chromosomes, which have been classified by geneticists into 23 consecutively numbered pairs. A mongoloid person, on the other hand, has 47 chromosomes in his cell nucleus. This ominous 47th chromosome is associated with the chromosome pairs 21 or 22. And precisely these pairs of chromosomes, in about

50 per cent of all people with chronic myeloid leukaemia, are altered in a remarkable way. One chromosome, in either pair 21 or 22, is halved.

It is astonishing that this mutilated "Philadelphia chromosome" is not found in other kinds of leukaemia. It is called the "Philadelphia chromosome" because it was discovered in Philadelphia.

An additional chromosome in mongolism, a missing half chromosome in leukaemia, both in the same pair of chromosomes, indicates a close relationship between leukaemia and mongolism. But perhaps there is also here a relationship which goes deeper into the puzzle of leukaemia, especially if the genes in these chromosomes should actually determine the growth of the white blood cells. If these genes should be damaged by X-rays, chemical substances or perhaps by viruses, then leukaemia could arise, or control of the growth of the white blood cells could be lost.

In other forms of cancer, too, the tragedy of the cell appears to begin in the innermost part of the nucleus. The road which led to this most common and convincing theory of the origin of cancer was long and littered with unavoidable errors. At the same time, it was a fascinating part of the history of human research and scientific knowledge.

Chapter 2

THE MAIN THEORIES

When a pathologist in the middle of last century examined cancerous tissue under the microscope, he could only discern the shape of the malignant cells. This outward form was the only apparent difference between healthy and malignant cells, and often it was not possible to differentiate clearly between harmless enlargements and malignant tumours.

The biochemical processes in the cell were still completely unknown; and the most important structures in the cell were still undiscovered. Only in 1831 was the cell nucleus discovered, and it was then merely known that the protoplasm, as it was called in the earliest textbook of general pathology, consisted of "an unprecedentedly complex mixture of proteins, fats and carbohydrates". Because man was consequently ignorant of the biochemical processes in the healthy cell, it was quite impossible to demonstrate differences in the malignant cells.

The pathologists of those times were certain of one thing: tumours of the same morphological type must consist of cells of the same kind, or at least of very similar cells. They considered each individual tumour as a homogeneous cell system. This concept of homogeneity was only disposed of by the results of research in recent decades. Today it is known that a single tumour consists of a whole mosaic of different cell types. The cells of such a tumour, which divide constantly, produce new cells that differ in their constitution and properties.

Even the familiar principle that cells arise exclusively from other cells was by no means general medical knowledge in the middle of the last century. Only in 1858 did Rudolf Virchow, one of the greatest medical men of his time, postulate, "Omnis cellula e cellula". Every cell arises from a cell. This was the eternal law of continuous development. According to Virchow, "the cell is the ultimate structural element of all living phenomena, both in health and disease, from which all the functions of life proceed".

The classical thesis of Virchow was of far-reaching significance in cell pathology and therapy. It was summed up 50 years later by Jacob Wolff, author of a history of cancer in the form of an encyclopaedia in 4 volumes. Wolff wrote: "All the earlier theories about the origin of cancer were eliminated."

The seat of life and death

Even earlier, in 1824, the French botanist Francois Vincent Raspail intuitively proclaimed: "If the cells are the seat of life and health, they must also be the seat of disease and death."

Cell-pathology was launched by Virchow, and the transition from humoral pathology to cell-pathology was completed.

Virchow also conceived the first scientifically based theory of cancer, in which the still fragmentary knowledge of the cell and its diseases was brilliantly interpreted.

This so-called theory of irritation is still valid to a limited degree for many present-day investigators of cancer. Virchow started from the thesis that a stimulus which acts on a cell for a long time, can cause that cell, through changes in its hereditary substance, to become malignant. The constantly irritated cell no longer conforms to its environment; it divides too rapidly and bequeaths its malignant properties to all of its daughter cells. Ultimately this leads to anarchistic communities in the cell-state, and to the formation of destructive tumours. The classification of solid tumours into different forms of cancer – such as carcinoma and sarcoma – also derives from Virchow.

Does tragedy begin in the uterus?

Two decades later, in 1878, there appeared another theory of cancer, which at once found many supporters. Julius Cohnheim, pathologist in Breslau and Leipzig, ascribed the origins of cancer to the organism of the foetus inside the uterus. In an early stage of embryonic development, cells are sometimes produced, so to speak, for storage. More are made than are needed for the development of the individual parts of the growing embryo.

Although the surplus may be trifling, embryonic cells have enormous capacities for growth and multiplication.

What happens when such immature cells, under certain influences, later seek quite suddenly to make up for time lost in their development?

Cohnheim thought that a cell catastrophe follows, for the delicately balanced regulators which control the differentiation of growth in the unborn organism, and stop it at the right times, are now absent, and the latent cells from the embryonic phase suddenly grow in unbridled fashion. They divide too rapidly, and finally become cancer cells.

This was, at the time, a very plausible explanation of the origin of cancer. Two undisputed facts seemed to support it. Embryonic malformations are, in fact, very common. These are not always the larger and conspicuous malformations caused by disturbance during the complex development from the fertilised egg to the completed organism, but may also appear in the microscopic sphere of the cell. There they lead to disturbances of the cell metabolism, and ultimately to metabolic diseases.

Among such malformations are so-called birth-marks, which occasionally give rise to very malignant tumours. A further basis for Cohnheim's theory, certain of great support among his pathologist colleagues, was the fact that the cells in many tumours show great similarity to embryonic tissues, or even organs.

Had Cohnheim actually found the key to the cancer problem? The scientific world discussed the question excitedly. But as more evidence was collected to support it, the more obvious its weaknesses became. As the French cancer investigator Charles Oberling wrote, "In order to explain the origin of malignant tumours, it was necessary to detect the existence of embryonic malformations. But such malformations are extremely common. Their number exceeds that of tumours many times over." There are, for example, moles. Almost everybody has several of these in the skin. But only very rarely do these pigment-forming cells produce malignant tumours. Thus one thing has been established: tissue malformations degenerate into cancer only in exceptional cases.

On the other hand, many scientists today consider it possible that there is a relationship between embryonic disturbances of growth and some kinds of tumour. Presumably these disturbances arise from damage to the respiration of the embryo, which finds too little oxygen in its environment. It seems that a result of this damage is that the doubling of the heredity material in the cell nuclei is prevented, for which reason many cells in the embryo die. If sufficient oxygen becomes available, the neighbouring cells try to make good the losses. Increased but unregulated cell multiplication sets in, and altered cells develop in certain parts of the embryo. These are the so-called "structural faults".

Professor Franz Büchner, formerly Pathologist in the University of Freiburg in Breisgau wrote: "Characteristic malformation of organs may arise in subsequent development from changes of this kind." Moreover there are in these "structural faults" cells which have not been fully differentiated and harbour a dangerous growth potential. Professor Büchner and other pathologists adopt the view that such cells – as Cohnheim once maintained – begin to grow much later on, and may then form tumours. Such structural damage may not only be caused by damage to the respiration of the cell, but also by radiation.

According to Büchner there is much to be said for the theory "that the most serious tumours of the brain, gliomas, are dysgenic in origin". In particular, brain tumours in children, which, next to leukaemia, are the second most common forms of cancer in juveniles, may be explained in this way.

The mystery of cell division

Millions of cells divide every second in the human body. But why is the division and growth of each of them adjusted to exactly the right moment, and why does the cancer cell alone lack this regulatory mechanism? This question, which persistently recurs in cancer research, drives the scientist to delve deeper and deeper into the mystery of cell life and the ritual of division. Cell division proceeds according to an unvarying biological schedule. It does not – as Virchow was the first to recognise – differ basically in the millions of living beings.

It is always the cell nucleus which begins the division – the mitosis. This nucleus floats in the plasma fluid of the cell. Theodor Schwann, one of the founders of the cell theory, still held it to be nothing more than "a structure composed of mucus and vegetable jelly", a reservoir for the stock piling of food materials.

Schwann was very much mistaken. The cell nucleus harbours not only the code for the specific reproduction of the entire heredity material, but also the control centre for thousands of processes in the remainder of the cell. It is therefore absolutely indispensable. A cell without a nucleus is incapable of living. It quickly and inevitably dies. If the nucleus is restored in time, the cell's "resurrection" begins: it returns to its normal activity.

The nucleus, with its chromosome apparatus, is undoubtedly the sovereign of the whole cell. It is not, to be sure, an absolute monarch. There are a number of indications that the cell plasma reacts in certain ways on the control mechanism in the nucleus. To put it in popular language, while the nucleus represents the "highest authority" in cell life, it nevertheless accepts "suggestions" which are made to it by the commanders in the cell province.

One can even speak of an interdependence between the nucleus and the cell plasma. At all events, this is indicated by recent research. Nuclei have been transferred from the cells of primitive organisms into plasma derived from more highly developed animals. This revealed the astonishing fact that, in this case, the cell nucleus also achieves a higher stage of development.

If cell respiration is damaged

An important part in this reciprocal influence and dependency is certainly played by the mitochondria. These were recognised shortly before the turn of the century as being regular constituents of the cell plasma. These tiny spherical or rod-shaped structures always collect within the cell at the sites in which the process of chemical manufacture is in full swing. They are like a kind of power station inside the cell, and play an important rôle in the oxidation processes in cell respiration. The enzymes stored in them help to break down the important foodstuffs in the cell, such as carbohydrates, fats and proteins, into smaller molecules. Only in this way can these be used by the cell for building up its structure.

Chemical substances and radiation, may injure these minute power houses and the enzymes which are so important for cell respiration. They stop the oxidation in the cell and convert oxidation into fermentation. The German biochemist and Nobel Prize Laureate Otto Warburg saw in this process the chief cause of the conversion of a normal cell into a cancer cell. As Warburg said, whilst the normal cell uses oxygen for respiration, the cancer cell gets its energy entirely from fermentation processes. Cancer as the result of damaged mitochondria and disturbed respiratory processes in the cell? The late Nobel Prize Laureate Gerhard Domagk said: "Our only hope lies along these lines," and the American cancer investigator Ernest L. Wynder stated in Berlin in 1965: "there will presumably not be any decisive advances in the treatment of this disease until the 'revitalisation' and restoration of the damaged mitochondria becomes possible."

Other experts completely reject this. Admittedly, as in all cancer theories, this one has too many exceptions. It is certain, for example, that not all cancer cells get their energy from fermentation, although this is true of most advanced tumours. Morover, many malignant cells show mitochondria that are absolutely intact. Yet another question is, at present, unanswered: how is the injury to the mitochondria, which is a defect in the cell plasma, passed on to the daughter cells? In the past, at least, it was difficult to understand how this could happen without the co-operation of the chromosomes, stationed in the nucleus. For the first time, a few years ago, the concept of intracellular feedback changed the biochemical view of life, and explanations of this phenomenon seem to be in sight.

A path through the cancer labyrinth

The most popular theory of the origin of cancer was conceived in 1928 in the train between Würzburg and Göttingen. In a railway compartment sat the young Doctor Karl Heinrich Bauer, reading the standard work "General pathology of malignant tumours", by the Munich pathologist Maximilian Borst. Bauer was once more impressed by the puzzling variety of human and animal tumours, as he had so often been while reading this book and in his own clinical experience. As this disease has so many aspects, he thought, must there not be somewhere in the cell nucleus a general release mechanism, a common factor to which the development of all kinds of cancer is related?

Bauer had been busy, not only with medical, but also with genetic and biological problems. He knew the modern work on spontaneous mutations in the germ cell and he had read with special attention the reports of the American geneticist, Hermann Joseph Muller, who was the first to succeed in producing mutations artificially in animals.

Muller's favourite material for research was the "domestic animal" preferred by geneticists, the fruit fly *Drosophila*. This fly reproduces itself rapidly and develops in a few days, so that 30 generations can be bred in one year. In addition, it possesses particularly large chromosomes. Even the individual heredity factors in these, the genes, are clearly visible under the microscope. Muller used this species to study mutations. First of all, he began to find out whether these mutations, the supposedly unintentional defects of heredity, are not also subject to certain laws.

In order to produce such defects in the gene material, Muller submitted the animals to harsh treatment. "They were" he reported, "poisoned, intoxicated, flooded with light, kept in the dark, half stifled by heat, stained inside and out, spun round and round, vigorously shaken, inoculated, mutilated and treated with everything there is".

All was useless. Muller could not produce any genetic changes. Nature had evidently taken every precaution to protect the genes in the chromosomes.

Muller then had to bring into action more powerful biological guns. Perhaps radiation would exert a more profound effect on the chromosomes. Muller therefore exposed the flies to an X-ray apparatus and irradiated them. Naturally he did not know how high a dose to give. Some flies promptly died; others were rendered infertile. But some of them remained fertile, and these were crossed with flies that had not been irradiated. Ten days later their descendants showed that mutations had appeared in their genes.

X-rays break up chromosomes

First calculations showed that irradiation had increased the mutation rate many times over. Microscopic investigation also showed that some of the chromosomes were even broken into pieces. "Here at last the Promised Land. The results of these experiments were sensational and unambiguous. The roots of life – the genes – were, in fact, stricken and they had given way."

In an article "Artificial transmutation of the gene" in 1927, Muller published for the first time the results of his mutation experiments on fruit flies, a discovery which gave an enormous stimulus to genetics and biochemistry and earned him the Nobel Prize.

In addition to X-rays, various chemical substances can produce mutations in germ cells. The researches of the German botanist Professor Friedrich Oehlkers in 1939, and the English Doctor Charlotte Auerbach in 1944, were epoch-making in this field of research. These two workers also used the fruit fly *Drosophila* for their experiments.

Charlotte Auerbach worked as a chemist during the Second World War on problems of chemical warfare. In this way she came to use in her mutation experiments the mustard gas that was so feared in the First World War. She was able to establish conclusively that mustard gas causes a breakdown in the cell nucleus and a rearrangement of the chromosomes. Mutations resulted in a considerable number of animals.

Meanwhile a long list of chemical substances with which humans come into daily contact had, in animal experiments, shown definite mutagenic effects.

When Bauer conceived his mutation theory, only a limited number of these genetic experiments had been carried out. They were concerned exclusively with mutations in the germ cells. But Bauer inferred, were not mutations in the body cells also conceivable? Does human cancer arise as a mutation, in which a normal body cell changes into a cancer cell and imprints on all its descendants the stamp of malignity?

After all, X-rays which cause mutations in germ cells, could cause cancer in body cells, as innumerable examples had shown. Mutations in germ cells and in body cells had one thing in common: they must have been caused by changes in the genes and chromosomes. Was this the secret of the fearful mechanism which changed a body cell into a cancer cell?

In favour of the mutation theory

"The birth of the mutation theory was the happiest hour of my life" confessed Bauer many decades later, at the celebration of his 75th birthday in the autumn of 1965. "I felt like a composer who has conceived the theme of his greatest work." The theme – cancer as the result of genetic changes in the body cells – also ran through the whole life work of surgeons and cancer research workers. Bauer could not provide any proofs of his theory, but there was much to be said for this new explanation of the cancerous process. The numerous and various influences which can cause cancer, whether they are X-rays, chemical substances or other factors, were all explained by it. Although carcinogenic factors are so numerous, they need only possess the common ability to cause mutations. If cancer arose through mutations in the body cells, the irrevocable nature of the change from normal to malignant cells could also be explained. Since a cancer cell can change to a certain extent, further, more malignant, mutations are possible – only it can, so to speak, no longer return to a "state of innocence". It can no longer become like its mother cells, before there was a genetic change.

But where does this genetic change occur inside the chromosomes?

When Bauer first formulated his theory, too little was known about the nucleic acids, deoxyribonucleic acid (DNA) in the cell nucleus, and ribonucleic acid (RNA) in the cell plasma. The universal part they play in the genetic process was still unsuspected, and it could not be foreseen that, within a few decades, they would become the subject of decisive studies by biochemists and molecular biologists. At the time when the mutation theory arose, it was only possible to suppose that mutations must affect the genes in the chromosomes. Important indications of this were the irregular chromosome structures which had already been detected in cancer cells.

A relationship no one thought of

Nobody thought of a connection between nucleic acid and cancer, or that these acids would one day provide the key to the cancer problem, although the first nucleic acid, deoxyribonucleic acid (DNA) was discovered in 1869, a good dozen years after Virchow had founded his cell theory. To be sure very little notice was taken of it in scientific literature. Yet the scientific findings of the Swiss chemist Friedrich Miescher, then just 26 years old, can be likened to the discovery of a hitherto unknown continent, even though it must have been more or less accidental and he was working only in the microscopic sphere.

Johann Friedrich Miescher was born in Basle on August 13, 1844. His father was Professor of Pathological Anatomy in the University there. The son studied medicine in the University of his home town and in Göttingen. He served his early scientific apprenticeship with the famous chemist Friedrich Wöhler in Göttingen, who, in 1828, was the first to succeed in synthesizing an organic substance, urea. Miescher's next and decisive appointment was in the Tübingen laboratory of Felix Hoppe-Seyler, one of the leading biochemists of his time; who is famous for his important researches on the functions of haemoglobin, the colouring matter of the red blood corpuscles.

Miescher discovers a new compound

Hoppe-Seyler had given the young Swiss chemist a task which in no way promised sensational discoveries. His pupil was to investigate the nuclei of animal pus cells. Miescher allowed a certain enzyme to act on these cells, namely the pepsin present in gastric juice, which plays a major part in breaking down protein molecules into smaller units during the process of digestion. The pepsin broke down the pus cells in such a way that their structure was dissolved and only the nuclei remained.

As Miescher analysed the nuclei, he found a hitherto completely unknown compound, which belonged neither to the carbohydrates, the fats or fat-like substances, nor to the sugars. Miescher had found it in the cell nucleus, so he christened it "nuclein".

No one today could say what impression this discovery made on the young Swiss chemist. He could certainly not anticipate that he had discovered the first clue to the greatest mystery of life, the basic chemical substance of all living things.

Hoppe-Seyler, Miescher's teacher, reacted to his pupil's report with understandable scepticism. Were there not many eventualities which deprived Miescher's discovery of any significance? Perhaps it was merely the result of impurities which had got in during the chemical analysis.

Soon Miescher went back to Basle and qualified there as a lecturer. A year later, when he was 28, he was appointed to the new Chair of Physiology in the University of Basle.

Now he renewed his study of nuclein. The chief supply of the nuclei required for this work came from salmon, which came in from the Atlantic and swam up the Rhine to the waterfalls just above Basle. In the sperm of these fish Miescher made a second great discovery. He isolated for the first time a group of animal proteins, the protamines, combined with the nucleic acid.

In addition he worked, using various organs of the Rhine salmon, on the significance of CO_2 tension as a respiratory stimulus and on the blood storage function of the spleen. His simultaneous research with his pupils on the influence of mountain climates on red blood cells laid the foundations of mountain-physiology. Then death put an end to his work; having suffered from lung tuberculosis for a year, he died in a sanatorium in Davos. He was then only 51.

Four years after Miescher's death, "Nuclein" was given its final name – nucleic acid – by the German scientist Richard Altmann, the discoverer of the mitochondria. The biochemist Albrecht Kossel, also a pupil of Hoppe-Seyler and later his assistant, continued Miescher's work on the chemistry of the cell nucleus. He analysed the basic kinds of protein obtained from nuclein and discovered the first chemical constituents of the nucleic acids.

In the shadow of the proteins

The precise part played by nucleic acids in the mechanism of heredity was still unknown. There was no great incentive for intensive study in this direction. For three-quarters of a century the nucleic acids were overshadowed, so to speak, by the proteins, which were held by most scientists to be much more interesting. Miescher's nuclein remained a kind of "Cinderella-compound", as an American investigator has called it. The knowledge that DNA forms the chemical substrate of the chromosomes and that the genes, so much discussed, were nothing more than DNA molecules, still lay in the far future.

After thirty years the "sleeping beauty" existence of the nucleic acids came to an end. A startling experiment by an English bacteriologist led for the first time to a conception of the almost fantastic function of DNA. It was in bacteria that Fred Griffith was able to discover that genetic characteristics were interchangeable and transmissible from one living being to another. This discovery of the transformation principle was a milestone in the history of genetic science. Further discoveries gradually revealed that the genetic material was none other than Miescher's DNA, the chemical link between generation and generation, the genetic code laid down in the cell as the biological law of development.

Griffith worked with pneumococci, which cause in man and animals a form of inflammation of the lungs. The bacteria are dangerous to man, or, for example, to mice, only because of their capsule. This consists of polysaccharides, long chains of certain sugar molecules – and it surrounds the interior of the bacteria. In this way it protects the bacterium from defensive agents developed by man and animals.

There are also, among the various types of pneumococcus, strains which have lost their ability to form capsules, and thereby their virulence. All the mice injected by Griffith with pneumococci from such strains remained free from infection. When they were exposed to encapsulated pneumococci which had been killed off by heat, the animals again showed no reaction. But when Griffith injected into his mice a mixture of strains without capsules and dead pneumococci with capsules, the result was completely different: after only a few days life ceased in the cages, the animals having wasted apathetically away. An examination of their blood revealed unquestionably the presence of encapsulated pneumococci.

Hereditary characteristics exchanged

The first thought was naturally that something must have gone wrong during the experiment. Perhaps, in some inexplicable way, a few of the encapsulated pneumocci had not been killed by the heat? But further investigations soon showed that this was not so: the encapsulated pneumococci were indubitably "clinically" dead. Now only one conclusion remained: in the dead encapsulated pneumococci there must be hidden a substance capable of transferring its hereditary characteristics to the pneumococci without capsules. What chemical substance could this be? Griffith supposed that it might be the polysaccharide itself which had caused the transformation which it soon became possible to demonstrate in the test tube.

Griffith's experiment meant the end of many earlier scientific theories. Accordingly, the response he received was at first sceptical. But for countless researchers throughout the world, it provided an immense stimulus. The whole of the next decade was taken up with further investigations into the substance capable of transmitting hereditable characteristics. And increasingly the evidence began to point in favour of DNA.

An American chemist who had previously been conducting research on immunity, was at first entirely sceptical about Griffith's work. His own experiments, however, very soon led to a confirmation of it, and even resulted in significant new progress.

Oswald T. Avery used two different strains of pneumococci. One of these had the ability to form capsules, whilst the other had lost it. As Director of a research group, Avery isolated from the encapsulated bacteria a substance on which he cultivated the associated bacteria which lacked capsules. As these pneumococci multiplied and divided, bacteria which lacked capsules were still found among their descendants. But others suddenly acquired capsules again and transmitted this characteristic anew. A genetic factor was responsible for the formation of a capsule, and had been transmitted from one kind of bacterium to the other.

With great difficulty Avery and his colleagues succeeded in obtaining this substance in a pure form and in crystallising it. Even after crystallisation it was genetically active.

The structure is determined

Further studies made it clear that this genetic factor was the long neglected DNA. At the same time they removed all doubt that DNA was the decisive substance of the chromosomes. Previously, it had been thought that the control of self-multiplication and of the biological interplay in the cell lay with the proteins that Miescher had also found in the chromosomes.

However, as soon as it was determined that this omnipotent function belonged to the DNA, biochemists began to seek out the constituents of this molecule of life and determine its actual structure. Already the German biochemist Albrecht Kossel had discovered two recurrent constituents of the DNA molecule; these were the bases adenine and guanine, which are purines. Later thymine and cytosine were also detected as components of DNA. These are pyrimidines.

These four constituents of the DNA molecule are usually designated by biochemists by their initials. Thus A. stands for adenine, T. for thymine, C. for cytosine and G. for guanine. The ABC of life is therefore amazingly brief. Each base in the DNA molecule is bound to sugar molecules, the so-called riboses. The compounds thus formed are called nucleotides and the nucleotides in the DNA molecules are respectively coupled together by phosphate groups.

The knowledge gathered by many investigators made it possible to determine the basic formula of the DNA molecule. But its actual structure remained undiscovered until 1952.

In that year a London group under the physicist Maurice Wilkins succeeded by means of radiology in explaining the three-dimensional structure of DNA. The diffraction pictures obtained by irradiation showed that the molecule had a regular three dimensional structure. It was always the same in all DNA molecules. The difference between individual molecules must therefore depend on the fact that the individual units within this generally valid structure were arranged differently.

The possible variants were demonstrated a year later by two investigators in the English University of Cambridge, the English physicist, Francis Crick and the American James Dewey Watson, then 24 years old, who had obtained a scholarship to study in European Universities and had gone first to Copenhagen and then to Cambridge.

Stimulated by the diffraction picture obtained by Wilkins, Crick and Watson succeeded in constructing a model of the DNA molecule, which was as daring as it was scientifically convincing. A popular image of it would resemble a long filiform and spirally twisted rope ladder. The ropes represent the ribose and phosphate groups. The rungs are composed of the four bases adenine, guanine, cytosine and thymine, in such a way that each rung consists of a pair of bases held together by hydrogen linkage.

It is important that only cytosine and guanine or adenine and thymine can combine to form a pair. Only the combinations, CG, GC, AT and TA are therefore possible. One such pair is hung, so to speak, on to the sugar-phosphate ropes.

Many molecular biologists also compare the structure of a DNA molecule to a spiral staircase. In this simile one pair of bases forms each of the steps. Millions of them must be accommodated in a single DNA molecule. The DNA chains present in every individual cell, placed end to end, measure about 1 metre; the DNA chains in all the cells of the human body make up an information tape about 16,000 million kilometres long. Geneticists with a taste for feats of calculation have estimated that the biological instructions stored up in this tape would provide a record that would play for 2.4 million years before it came to an end.

"The technician," declared the Tübingen molecular biologist, Prof. G. Schramm, "who is accustomed to using tape recorders or calculating machines for storing information, will be astonished at the small space in which Nature stores great quantities of information. It can be calculated that the building plans for every human now living can be housed in a drop of nucleic acid smaller than a thimble."

Schramm's question as to "how blue prints co-ordinated with one another in the minutest detail have got into the nucleic acids" leads us into the realms of metaphysics. "It is certain they do not come from a human mind. On the contrary, it must be assumed that man as a rational being originated in accordance with the instructions present in the molecules."

Schramm supposes that since all living beings developed from simple evolutional states, the nucleic acids must also have been formed at some point in the earth's history. In his laboratory a simple method was found to produce nucleic acids of high molecular weight in a non-biological way. "Admittedly, the nucleotides in these synthetic nucleic acids are still completely disordered. But we see," hoped Schramm "certain possibilities of imitating in the test-tube the process of storing and increasing information."

American scientists have already produced nucleic acids biochemically. In 1956, the American biochemist and Nobel Laureate Arthur Kornberg "built" the first artificial DNA chain with the aid of enzymes. In this process a little DNA is required as a "starter". A year earlier Kornberg's colleague S. Ochoa – an American of Spanish descent – had made a short chain of ribonucleic acid units with the help of an enzyme taken from bacteria. For this work, he, too, received the Nobel Prize.

RNA is chemically closely related to DNA. Its sugar contains one more oxygen atom. Instead of thymine, RNA has the nitrogenous base uracil. To all appearances RNA is formed from DNA by a kind of off-print from the DNA mould. Subsequently the RNA is discharged from the nucleus into the cell plasma to guide the formation of proteins.

No animal or plant could exist without these proteins: they are the most important basic substance of the muscles and blood (the antibodies present in the blood, which protect the body against foreign invaders such as bacteria or viruses, also consist of proteins).

Enzymes, too – or ferments as they are also called – are chemically nothing but proteins. They are, to be sure, mostly of significantly more complex structure than the simple body proteins. Without these bio-catalysts the innumerable chemical reactions that go on in the cell would not function – because many chemical reactions in cells do not occur spontaneously, or at any rate not quickly enough.

The genetic code is deciphered

Proteins are made up of amino acids – their succession is in turn determined by the sequence of the bases in the ribonucleic acid molecule. Because there are about 20 different amino-acids, the four nucleic acid bases are insufficient for the formulation of the secret code. A combination of nucleotides must thus be responsible for the making of an amino acid. Mathematically it follows that one pair of combinations is not enough, because in this way only 16 amino acids could be determined. Molecular biologists therefore assume that three nucleotides respectively, a triplet, constitute the code for one amino acid. Numerous experiments seem to establish that this assumption is correct.

In America a large part of this secret code has been successfully deciphered. It has been established which base units determine various amino acids. For this purpose synthetic nucleotides were used. Dr Marshal Nirenberg, a young American biochemist, was the first to make an artificial RNA.

This RNA contained only one organic base, uracil. Then he added this synthetic RNA, with the three code-units, to a mixture of various amino acids. Which of these amino acids would respond to the synthetic RNA and unite to form a protein? Because the RNA contained only a single cue, it could be only one of the amino acids present. The experiment gave a clear answer. The result was a protein exclusively composed of phenylalanine.

In this way the first letter, so to speak, in the genetic code was revealed: three times U signified nothing else but phenylalanine. Later Nirenberg and other investigators used this system to determine, little by little, the units of the code – or base triplets as they are also called – for almost all the amino acids. In this way it was often found that the same amino acid can be determined by several triplets.

Of course, a complete sequence analysis of the RNA has not so far been possible, so that up to now the results permit only a statistical interpretation. It was possible to deduce which kinds of base were respectively responsible for the formation of an amino acid. The sequence in which the bases in the RNA and DNA molecule are arranged cannot be analysed by the scientific methods at present available.

But one day perhaps it will be possible to determine the genetic material of a bacterium embodied in the secret chemical code, i.e. to describe each single section of the DNA molecule. Such a sequence analysis of the DNA of human cells is also conceivable. This would necessitate immense advances not only in molecular biology itself, but also in electronics and other sciences.

In addition to the messenger RNA, which transports the control and building plans of DNA into the cell plasma, a second RNA takes part in the complex team work of protein synthesis. This so-called transfer-RNA contains the same code units, and sees to it that the necessary amino acids are united in the right sequence. The individual amino acids are arranged end to end by the transfer-RNA, in the right position on the conveyor belt of the messenger-RNA for the making of protein.

RNA from yeast

The structure of a transfer RNA was determined for the first time not long ago. In 1957 a young chemist, Dr. Robert Holley, began work in this direction in a laboratory of the American Ministry of Agriculture in Cornell University.

Previously Holley had isolated from simple baker's yeast a transfer RNA which carried the amino acid alanine to the "building site" of the protein synthesis in the yeast cell. Unfortunately this alanine-transfer RNA was still quite impure. It had to be isolated in a much purer form before Holley could devote himself to the task which he had set himself: the determination of its structural formula.

In 1959, Holley's Cornell Laboratory team began work with enormous quantities of yeast. A hundred pounds of yeast at a time were mixed with about 90 litres of phenol and 135 litres of water. By this method the team obtained from 300 lb. of yeast about 200 grammes of impure Transfer-RNA.

After 3 years Holley succeeded in obtaining, from this 200

grammes, just 1 gramme of the pure substance. He and his colleagues worked for another 3 years with this small quantity until, in the middle of 1965, it was possible to elucidate the structural formula of alanine-transfer RNA. To do this, two different enzymes were used, which broke down the RNA in various sequences of smaller pieces, so-called rows of nucleotides. It was then possible to analyse these pieces, so that ultimately the task remaining for the research team was to put together the individual formulae, like a jig-saw puzzle.

In this way it was discovered that alanine-transfer RNA consists of 77 nucleotides with a combined molecular weight of about 26,600. Nine of these nucleotides did not belong to the usual constituents of RNA molecules and had been previously completely unknown. In spite of its complex polymer structure, this transfer-RNA certainly belongs to the simplest nucleic acids, because in most other RNA molecules several thousand nucleotides are contained in a single molecule.

The enthusiasm with which scientists welcomed this first structural explanation of an RNA as a milestone in research, is, however, justified. When the structure of the various nucleic acids is known, the basis is provided for the investigation of the functions of the nucleic acids and ultimately for their synthesis. After successful syntheses doctors could finally hope for the specific treatment of many diseases caused by genetic faults of development. Among these are symptoms of lack of hormones, forms of muscular dystrophy and especially some forms of cancer.

Holley's group has already obtained in pure form two other kinds of transfer-RNA and is working on the elucidation of their structural formulae. Dr. Richard D. O'Brien, Director of the biochemical division of Cornell University, estimates that 10–20 years will be needed for the elucidation of the structure of all the nucleic acids present in the DNA-RNA complex. But then, he thinks, it should be possible to "manipulate" the genetic material for a whole series of useful purposes, from the modification of plants and animals, which are important for human nutrition, to the control of genetic faults in development and of diseases which are connected with DNA.

"Misprints" in the genetic code

Nucleic acids as the key substance of life, but also the key to two great conceptions of disease! This is how the American

Nobel Prize Laureate Linus Pauling saw the situation, when he coined the expression "sick molecule". On the one hand, there are the genetic diseases. They arise from changes in the DNA in the hereditary substance, and can be transmitted by reproduction from generation to generation. On the other hand, there are diseases caused by changes in the DNA of the body cells.

Cancer undoubtedly belongs to this latter category. It has often been described as a misprint in the genetic code. "We consider cancer to be a genetic disease at the cellular or perhaps the molecular level, which reflects changes in the architecture of the nucleic acids. This is the basic idea and theme of our research work," said Dr. Aaron Bendich, head of the biochemical division of the Sloan-Kettering Institute, in which he has worked since 1947. "In those days" he said, "the suspicion arose that the nucleic acids must have something to do with cancer. This suspicion has since become an absolute certainty."

In his view the DNA of a cancer cell must be different from that of a normal cell. But what kind of difference could this be? Is a genetic component lost in division, does a defect occur in the self-multiplication, or is a new piece of genetic information added to the DNA? Perhaps by a carcinogenic virus?

Bendich went for the third possibility. In support of it he isolated the DNA of the carcinogenic polyoma-virus and transferred it to cultures of normal mouse cells. There the DNA caused exactly the same morbid cell changes as the intact virus did. When these cultures were injected into newly-born hamsters, they developed tumours.

This experiment, noted throughout the world, showed clearly that pure DNA could cause cancer. But it was still not proved that the DNA added new genetic material to the cell. In order to decide this Bendich marked DNA, from the white blood cells of man, with a radioactive hydrogen isotope and added this marked material to human cells bred in a tissue culture. These were the so-called Hela cells, obtained decades ago from an American woman with cancer of the uterus and subsequently cultivated for many generations.

The first stage of this research was successful. The marked DNA actually penetrated into the cell nucleus and could clearly be detected there, as Bendich and his collaborator Dr. Ellen Borenfreund were able to record.

"Now," concluded Bendich, "we must find out whether and how the carcinogenic virus penetrates into the chromosomes. That is one of the most important questions that we are now studying." If there should one day be a positive answer, innumerable further problems will arise. How can the infinitely long sequences of a DNA molecule – estimated to be several millions – be analysed? How can the DNA-portions of a healthy cell be compared with those of a cancer cell? How can we alter certain pairs of bases or even single atoms in DNA, in order to find out what such procedures cause, and whether they can possibly lead to cancer cells?

Germ cells and body cells react differently

Although biochemistry and molecular biology have advanced at such a tremendous rate in recent years, we must at present expect there to be many years of further research before the DNA molecule is "in the bag". Then it will be possible for the first time to reach a definite conclusion about the mutation theory, which is based upon the changes in these genetic structures. Until then, many scientists will continue to oppose Bauer's conjecture on the grounds that mutations in the body cells, in contrast to those in the germ cells, are not detectable.

Bauer is well armed to counter this criticism. It does not take account – he says – of the fundamental difference between germ cells and body cells. How could both kinds of cell react in the same way, asks Bauer, if they are fundamentally different in nature? Germ cells have single sets of chromosomes and body cells doubled ones; germ cells act as individual cells, body cells in tissue associations; germ cells are designed to build up the whole organism, body cells are already differentiated and have special tissue functions; germ cells are concerned with reproduction and body cells with metabolism.

These are important differences, so one cannot expect, says Bauer, that factors which cause cancer in body cells will always cause mutations in germ cells. In spite of all the objections to it, the mutation theory remains impressive: it introduces a line of direction into the bewildering labyrinth of cancer. If the origin of cancer is interpreted as a mutation then even Virchow's old irritation theory is, according to Bauer, viewable in a new light. The Berlin "Pontiff of medicine" had – as has already been mentioned – formulated in the middle of last century a modern theory of cancer, which took into account all the knowledge of cell life gained through the light microscope. Virchow thought that cells and tissues which are exposed for a long time to chronic irritation would react by rapid division, and would ultimately become malignant.

But the 60 billion or so cells of the human body do not divide in a constant manner. There is only a limited truth in the often-quoted phrase that the human body renews itself every seven years, since this is the time it would take for all the cells to replace themselves. Some tissues, in fact, renew themselves continuously; others cannot do this at all. At the birth of a human being, all the nerve and muscle cells are already formed. They fulfil their tasks for as long as the individual lives. If a nerve cell is destroyed, it is irreparable. A nerve cell that has been differentiated can no longer divide, and the body does not possess a "stock" of nerve cells.

Between 1 per cent and 2 per cent of human cells die day by day. Thus in the human body there are areas of active cell-change, especially in the tissues of the skin, in the blood cells, in the digestive organs and the sex glands. Other organs are renewed much less often.

Many cells are, in fact, capable of division but need a special stimulus to divide. Professor K. H. Bauer writes: "For subscribers to the mutation theory, 'chronic irritation' thus acquires a new and correct sense." In this context, the decisive question is whether chronic irritation stimulates resting cells to new and continued divisions, and thus starts a process of hypertrophy. In normal tissues this would clearly not lead to tumour formation; in this Virchow was wrong.

A different picture could result if a cell which was exposed to a somatic mutation were continuously irritated. So long as it does not divide, it does not produce any malignant descendants. It is isolated and therefore harmless. But if such a cell is suddenly incited to new divisions, then it may impress the stamp of cancer on later cell generations, until enough of its kind have arisen to form a tumour and to start a general attack in the human body.

Another explanation of cancer also acquired a new aspect through the mutation theory. This was the regeneration theory, propounded by Professor Bernhard Fischer-Wasels, formerly pathologist at Frankfurt University. Fischer-Wasels started from the fact that cancer chiefly breaks out in a cell-tissue which suffers continual injury and damage. It is therefore found in regeneration that is constant and often disturbed. Where the tissues that divide are particularly active, there is always a certain risk. The more actively the cells divide, the earlier may mutations, and ensuing malignant degeneration, occur. Embryonic cells are also especially sensitive to the influence of mutations. Their hereditary substance can be damaged by extremely small doses of radiation or chemical substances. Numerous injuries in different chromosomes offer clear proof of this.

A series of mutagenic events

Bauer's mutation theory received powerful backing from the immunologist Sir Frank Macfarlane Burnet. The Australian Nobel Prize Laureate expressed the opinion in 1959 that cancer cells arise by a "series of mutagenic events". Burnet would clearly be most pleased if the terms "mutagenic" and "carcinogenic" were always identical. His interpretation of the course of the cancerous process is as follows: the first cancer cells caused by mutagenic events form a smaller collection of cells, from which the tumour then develops. But it is still necessary that these malignant cells have a "proliferative advantage" over the healthy cells. A special hormonal influence for example, could, promote such growth or hypertrophy.

The well-known American investigator, Van Rensselaer Potter, also came out in favour of the mutation theory in 1958. Cancer, Potter thought, can be considered as a "developmental problem in a blind-alley". At the end of it stands death for both host and cancer cells, brought about by an error in the doubling of the DNA in the prophase of division.

Nucleic acids must not make errors

In the multiplication of DNA, the two halves of the molecule separate. Subsequently each strip recreates itself, by means of the nucleotides present in the cell, into a new and complete double strip, which is an accurate copy of the original one. Because each of the giant molecules of DNA consists of an infinitely variable succession of millions of pairs of bases, errors in the production of the genetic code are conceivable.

Scientists estimate that this can occur perhaps once in 10 million cases. Irradiation or chemical substances can greatly increase the frequency of such a molecular mishap, but because the cell contains only a limited stock of nucleotide building components, there is a limit to the number of possible mutations.

Present scientific methods clearly cannot prove that cancer arises from a spontaneous change in the DNA. Professor Hans Lettré, for example, one of the foremost German investigators of cancer, will neither admit or deny such a possibility. On the other hand, such "innate errors" of the DNA would explain the frequency of cancer. For there is no doubt that previous damage due to radiation or chemical substances can only be found in the smallest number of cancer patients. To give only one example: cancer of the lung is, for many scientists, the standard example of exogenous causes. But why do people suffer from lung cancer who never smoke or who have never been exposed to the atmospheric impurities of large towns and industrial establishments? To this there has so far been no satisfactory answer.

It is obvious that cancer is not caused by every mutation of the body cells. Professor Lettré said that "the normal cell can only react to injuries which do not actually kill it with a limited number of evasive measures. One of them is the cancer cell." The disease probably only has a chance when certain nucleic acid molecules, or pieces of DNA, which are responsible for the social integration of the cells, are affected. Nobody yet knows which parts of the nucleic acids are able to do this.

Genes are switched on and off

Perhaps the genes which guide protein synthesis are not the primary target of cancer agents in every instance. In recent years, the classical concept of the gene has been broadened. In addition to the normal gene, the individual genetic factor, scientists now postulate the existence of other kinds. For example, regulator genes, which are responsible for switching the structure-genes on and off and thus determining the areas of information in the DNA sections to be set free for protein synthesis. To increase the variety still further: the regulator-genes in turn depend upon special operator-genes which activate the structure-genes. Scientists were first led to this conception of the "trinity" of genetic apparatus by the fact that the store of information in the DNA of each of the various tissue cells contains the plan for the construction of the whole organism. But a nerve cell, liver cell or brain cell needs only a fraction of this information. The rest of it is "censored" by other genes or nucleic acid units.

The need for enzymes and protein also varies in the different phases of cell life. It can therefore be assumed that many genes are permanently or temporarily switched off. Andre Lwoff, Professor of Microbiology in the Sorbonne, Paris, and one of the three Nobel Laureates in 1965, was the first to show, in bacteria infected with a virus, that whole gene complexes can be put out of action for generations.

It is believed that mutations occur directly in those regulator-genes which control the action of the operator genes. If this control is abolished the operator genes are, so to speak, let off the leash; the genes which have become "sick" may then begin to run amok, and the collapse of growth control may begin.

Possibly the DNA is also subjected to another control authority. Friedrich Miescher, the discoverer of the nucleic acids, had already shown that cell nuclei contain a certain protein in addition to DNA. Later this was called histone. It seems to mask part of the DNA sequences, so that only the desired portion of the DNA information can be read off by the messenger RNA – which is responsible for protein synthesis.

It has been found that many tumour cells contain an unusually high content of histone in their nucleus. The tumour cells would thus be supplied with less information and therefore would not be able to observe the laws of cell life. Still more probable would be the reverse mechanism, namely, a lack of histone – perhaps caused by carcinogens – as a result of which too much information was released and control of growth arrested.

If this admittedly speculative conception is allowed, there are two different possibilities of the genesis of tumours: a direct effect on the nucleic acids or on the controlling action of the histone.

Mutations in the cell plasma

Not all cancer investigators and microbiologists subscribe to the thesis that the first step in the disaster of cancer must occur in the hereditary structures in the cell nucleus. Professor Arnold Graffi, speaking of researches in the Paul Ehrlich Institute in Frankfurt-am-Main, expressed the view in 1939 that cancer could also occur under certain conditions as the result of a mutation outside the nucleus.

Graffi, now chief of the Cancer Research Institute of the

Academy of Science in East Berlin, wished at that time to find out how carcinogenic hydrocarbons are distributed in tissues and cells. To do this, he dropped benzpyrene on the skin of mice and examined tissue samples under the fluorescent microscope, which can detect very small quantities of the hydrocarbon.

Graffi was surprised to find that the benzpyrene was stored preferentially in the cell plasma and especially in the mitochondria. This carcinogenic substance was, on the other hand, scarcely discernible in the nucleus. This suggested that mutation processes which transformed a healthy cell into a cancer cell might also occur in the mitochondria.

The English zoologist and geneticist Cyril Dean Darlington, of Oxford University, came to similar conclusions in 1948. Darlington also thought it possible that a kind of gene may be hidden in the cell plasma, constituting hereditary structures outside the nucleus.

It was known that the mitochondria, which look, under the electron microscope, like tiny sausage-shaped particles, play an important part in the metabolism of the cell. They serve as a kind of reservoir of enzymes and contain the most important ferments for the combustion of food substances and for the supply of energy in the cell. It was, however, difficult to conceive how it should be possible for the mitochondria to transmit genetic information, because the DNA necessary for this had, at the time, been found only in the cell nucleus.

"I saw" Graffi recollects today, "almost all my hopes float away". But the situation suddenly changed, when DNA was discovered in the mitochondria. The chief credit for this was due to the Swedish husband and wife research team K. & S. Nass, working in Philadelphia, and to the Belgian M. Chèvremont.

As Graffi emphasizes, "A gate was suddenly opened which led into new fields of research. Studies of the mitochondria are now also the chief field of research in our Institute." The Austrian scientist E. Wintersberger, and later Graffi also, were able to establish that, apparently with the help of the DNA in the mitochondria, ribonucleic acid is also synthesized. "Thus," says Graffi, "there is a possibility that the mitochondria represent points of attack by carcinogens."

When defective mitochondria are investigated, the chief emphasis should in future not only be placed on defects in the respiratory system. Abnormal manifestations in protein metabolism are also of great significance. "We assume" says Graffi, "that mutations are produced by the effects of carcinogens on the mitochondria. These lead, so far as we can perceive, to a reduction in protein synthesis. The ratio between protein and DNA shifts in the mitochondria of tumour cells in favour of the DNA, and we have been able to discover an increased quantity of DNA in tumour mitochondria. This greater amount of DNA is also found in a comparison between mitochondria in tumour cells and those in healthy, rapidly-growing tissues, which is of special importance in an investigation of the conditions in cancer cells." Such genetic changes in the cell plasma would only be a "necessary extension" of the mutation theory, Graffi explained in a conference in Heidelberg in 1965.

Feedback in the cell

At present, plasma genes are only one of the many tracks in the new country of biochemistry that cancer investigators have followed. Perhaps they are no more than biological phantoms. On the other hand, if they actually exist and if there is biologically active DNA in the mitochondria, then their relationship to the cancer process must be elucidated.

Yet another possibility is nowadays discussed in relation to the first point of attack by cancer. A hypothesis which has only recently been presented depends on the newly developed conception of feed-back mechanism. The American cancer investigator Potter wrote: "Whilst the conception of the gene consolidates our knowledge of evolution, the concept of feedback consolidates our knowledge of adaptation." Not only are there feedback mechanisms between different organ systems, for instance in the hormonal interplay of the body, but it must be assumed that they are also very probable in the interior of the cell.

When considering a feedback system, special attention should be given to those kinds of carcinogens which act not on the cell nucleus with its DNA structures, but on the cell plasma. In this way, not only will cell-specific protein be reduced, but the sites of protein synthesis will be attacked directly.

When these sites fail, the cell nucleus reacts with an overproduction of messenger RNA, which is discharged into the cell plasma. But there this messenger acid is altered by the carcinogenic substances. Then, by retroaction through this altered

RNA, changes occur in the DNA in the nucleus. This falsified information is transmitted afresh by DNA reproduction to the hereditary substance of newly-formed cells.

A result of this very complex process, which presumes various forms of interplay between the cell nucleus and the cell plasma, would be an indirect mutation. The Freiburg pathologist Franz Büchner wrote: "the restrictions on growth normally secured, in the course of differentiation, by the feedback between specific protein and DNA, thus lose their efficacy. The result is a continuous replication of DNA and an incessant cell-growth in the commencing and advancing carcinoma." Büchner saw in this thesis, which is also advocated by Professor Wolfgang Oehlert of Freiburg, no antagonism to the mutation theory. On the contrary it "gives significant precision" to Bauer's theory which thus becomes much more probable.

Chapter 3

THE SEARCH FOR CAUSES

If cancer is one day conquered, it will be thanks to millions of animals which have died in the course of research. The little that man knows today about the cause of cancer is due to innumerable researches on rabbits, rats, hamsters and many other animals. Cancer investigators all over the world require about a million mice alone every year.

Tumours in these animals are induced by new chemical substances, by radiation and virus infections. Minute pieces of tissue from these tumours are transplanted into other animals, and in this way the malignant cell-growth is studied in all the laboratories of the world. New weapons are tested on animals, and through them we strive to master the original disease. Imperfect as chemotherapeutic substances against cancer might be, even they would not be available to clinicians were they not tested by protracted experiments on animals.

If one studies the history of this disease over the centuries, it is clear that it was not animals, but men who were the first involuntary subjects of cancer research, and who provided scientists with the first indications that a fatal relationship must exist between certain chemical substances and cancer.

Chimney-sweep's disease

In 1775, the distinguished London surgeon Sir Percival Pott broke a limb, and so finally found the time to write a book he had long contemplated. Pott included in it some pages on a type of malignant tumour that he had often observed in his practice: cancer of the scrotum.

Mainly middle-aged men were affected by these tumours, and Pott found that almost all of them had worked when young as "climbing boys". Only children of 8 to 10 years old were able to force themselves through the narrow and winding chimneys of the English middle class houses of that time, and many of these juvenile chimney sweeps later acquired painful tumours which were the prelude to long illness and early death. Pott declared "the fate of these people seems to be incomparably harsh. In their early youth they are often treated with great brutality; they are exposed to cold and hunger; they are sent up narrow chimneys that are often still hot, they are scalded, burned and half suffocated. And when they become adults a cruel, painful and fatal disease awaits them . . ."

Soot as a cause of cancer

But what could have caused this disease and why were chimney-sweeps especially affected by it? No one knew; Pott often puzzled over this question, until ultimately the suspicion came to him that it must have been the soot, ground into the skin of the scrotum from the boys' clothes, which later caused the malignant tumours. Further observations strengthened this vague supposition, so that Pott was ultimately able to establish that "this disease undoubtedly originates in the professional occupation of the young chimney sweeps" – a statement which has become part of the history of cancer.

This was the first clear picture of a vocational cancer. It is not the only one. During the industrial revolution of the second half of the last century, additional categories of vocational cancer were soon recorded. Most of them were skin cancers since the skin most often, and most usually, comes into direct contact with substances that cause cancer. And these types of cancer are most easily discovered. It became possible, for example, to show that in addition to soot, the paraffin and arsenical compounds used in various branches of industry are other causes of cancer.

The Frankfurt urologist, Ludwig Rehn, ferreted out another vocational cancer. In this the relationship between the carcinogenic substance and the organ affected was not at first so obvious. This was cancer of the bladder, which was naturally not new to Rehn.

The cause of it was just as unknown as was that of other kinds of cancer. When three workmen suffering from cancer of the bladder came to Rehn's clinic – all of whom were employed in the same factory, Rehn sensed that he might have a clue. Could chemical substances, with which these patients were occupied, have caused their cancer?

The men worked for a firm which made pigments. Among these was fuchsin red, a brilliant dye-stuff needed by the rising textile industry. This substance was apparently a fatal risk for the workers. In an article in the "Archiv für Klinische Chirurgie" and at the Surgical Congress of 1895, Rehn expressed the opinion that these tumours of the bladder might be traceable to the aniline used in the pigments.

Rehn was thus the first to discover a cancer of an internal organ caused by external chemical poisons. Rehn's observations were soon strengthened by reports from other countries in which a dye-stuff industry had been established. In the course of time it became clear that this "aniline cancer" is not caused by the aniline itself, but by certain aromatic amines, such as betanaphthylamine or benzidine.

A decisive experiment

In these first forms of chemically induced cancer, human beings were the involuntary subjects of experiment. Two Japanese scientists were the first to succeed in causing cancer in animals by means of chemical substances. In the past, all experiments of this kind had failed; it was later shown that early investigators had not exposed their animals to the chemical carcinogens for long enough.

But the two Japanese, Yamagiwa and Itchikawa, had almost inexhaustible patience. Whilst Europe resounded with war alarms, the two investigators worked calmly on their cancer experiments. For months they painted tar on the insides of rabbits' ears. They chose this spot to exclude any confusion with spontaneous tumours. After two to three months, wart-like growths appeared in the animals, ulcers with hardened edges which ultimately became actual tumours.

After the rabbits, mice were treated with chemical substances. They were even more sensitive to carcinogens. Nowadays, chemically-induced tumours, in addition to transplanted and tissue-cultivated cancer cells are the stock in trade of every investigator of cancer.

Pott saw in the tarry constituents of soot the cause of cancer of the scrotum. The German doctor, Richard von Volkmann, discovered in 1875 "tar cancer" in workers who had to do with tar products. Ultimately it was established that cancer is also caused by tar in rabbits and mice. Now, in the 1920's cancer investigators conducted intensive studies of tar, which is clearly a mixture of hundreds of different chemical compounds.

To find the carcinogenic substances in this diffuse mixture was like seeking a needle in a haystack. Gradually it became clear that hydrocarbons with several rings in their chemical constitution were most likely to be the substances looked for. But there were innumerable modifications of these in tar, and they were only contained in the fractions with a higher boiling point, as Bruno Bloch, the Zürich investigator had proved.

A few milligrams suffice . . .

An English research group led by Sir Ernest Kennaway, of the London Cancer Hospital, ultimately won this marathon race of investigators. In 1932 they succeeded in isolating, from about 40 barrels of coal tar, a substance present in the tar only to the extent of 0.003 per cent – 3, 4 benzpyrene, one of the most dangerous carcinogens. As Sir Ernest said later: "the fluorescence spectrum was the vital aid which led us through this labyrinth." It had been found that the carcinogenic tars were all strongly fluorescent, and that their fluorescence spectrum showed three characteristic bands in the region of 4,000 Ångstroms.*

The decisive indication for the London research group was the discovery that some hydrocarbons show a similar spectrum. Among these is 1, 2 benzanthacene, which also causes cancer. By working on this, they finally produced 3, 4 benzpyrene. Doses of a few millionths of a gram of this are enough to cause cancer in animals. If the animals are painted with it, cancer of the skin develops, and if it is injected under the skin of mice or rabbits, sarcomas are formed.

* This unit of measurement is named after the Swedish physicist Anders Jöns Ångstrom, who taught in the previous century in the University of Uppsala. One Ångstrom (Å) means a length of one hundred millionth of a centimetre.

The results obtained by Kennaway and his colleagues naturally posed a new question: to what extent is there a relationship between the carcinogenic activity of these substances and their chemical constitutions? Kennaway, and his pupils were occupied for decades with this question.

Their main research materials were the carcinogenic hydrocarbons, which represented about half of the 450 known chemical carcinogens. But, despite the scientists' prolongued study of hydrocarbons, little is yet known about how they act. As Professor Eric Boyland complained in a speech in the London Chester Beatty Institute, "We know less about them than about many other chemical carcinogens which were discovered considerably later". Presumably this is due to the fact that hydrocarbons first pass through a series of changes in the body. They only become carcinogens by means of the body's help.

Target for attack: the DNA

Another group of carcinogenic substances attacks the hereditary substances directly, i.e. the DNA in the cell nucleus. These are the alkalysing substances, a quite different group of organic chemicals. The most important of them are nitrogen-mustard compounds (mustard gas), epoxide, ethylenimine, methan sulphonate or certain lactones. They add an alkyl group, i.e., a hydrocarbon group, to substances on which they act. In the germ cells of animals they cause grave genetic changes, and in body cells they can cause cancer. At the same time, they can inhibit the growth of transplanted tumours in animals – being carcinogens and cancer-inhibitors in one.

Such a class of compounds deserves the closest attention. Once again it was Professor Eric Boyland and Sir Alexander Haddow who took up the study. In 1949 they were able to report about the various mustard gas compounds which caused tumours in animals when injected either subcutaneously or intravenously.

During the next decade many other alkalysing substances were tested in cancer laboratories. Ethylenimine, teramine and diepoxide clearly showed a carcinogenic effect in animals. But an alkalysing substance is, generally speaking, a less powerful carcinogen than the polycyclic hydrocarbons.

As has been said, hydrocarbons presumably become carcinogenic through chemical reconstruction in the cell. Alkalysing substances on the other hand act more directly; they attack the DNA itself and deform the "molecule of life".

But at present there is no method of clearly detecting changes in or loss of DNA-sequences. Presumably alkalysing substances, which readily enter into combinations, influence not only the DNA but also the RNA and the cell proteins. Wherever cancer investigators may see the first point of attack of carcinogenesis, in the DNA in the cell nucleus, in the RNA or other structures in the cell plasma, they all find clear evidence for their conception among the alkalysing substances.

The hypothesis that cancer cells evade growth control because certain cell proteins are absent from them, has been shown by experiment. The American couple Elizabeth and James Miller, of the University of Wisconsin, treated rats in 1947 with the carcinogen 4-dimethylaminoazobenzene (butter-yellow). In this way they were able to observe that part of the carcinogen had a marked effect on the liver proteins of these animals. Subsequently, tumours developed which lacked proteins normally present in healthy liver tissue. The two investigators therefore concluded that this loss of protein, which inhibited growth, must be a decisive factor in the process of malignity.

Later investigations showed that other kinds of carcinogens combine with cell proteins. But this effect is also produced by substances which are not carcinogenic. Therefore the hypothesis of loss of protein lost ground some years ago.

Because every cancer cell transmits its malignant properties – the American investigator Dr. Jacob Furth was able to cause a tumour by injecting a single cancer cell into an animal – direct interference by the chemical carcinogen with genetic substances in the nucleic acid seemed most probable. Such combinations with nucleic acids have been detected not only with the aromatic amines, the azo-dyes, but also with the nitroso-compounds.

Liver tumours caused by nitrosamines

Nitroso-compounds appear to act in an alkalysing manner. In 1950 it was discovered in British laboratories that they can cause cancer; this was after dimethylnitrosamine had been used for many years as an apparently harmless solvent in the chemical industry of Great Britain. It served as an intermediate product in the manufacture of medicines and rocket propellants. But then two employees in a factory which produced this compound became ill with an obscure disease of the liver. The firm asked the distinguished Medical Research Council to investigate the matter. Using experiments on animals, the two scientists P. N. Magee and J. M. Barnes proved that nitrosamine can, in fact, cause liver disease and malignant tumours.

Such results were bound to alarm those working in industrial and academic research. All the derivatives of nitrosamine have therefore been carefully tested recently on many species of animals. Professor Hermann Druckrey in Freiburg, one of the most distinguished German investigators of cancer, did a great deal of work with nitrosamines. In a series of papers he proved that nitrosamine tumours can start in quite different parts of the body. Apparently it depends on which nitrosamine derivative is used whether gastric, liver or brain tumours develop.

The site at which the tumour develops seems to depend on the hydrocarbon group to which the amino-nitrogen of the nitrosamine is attached. If, for example, the nitrosamine of methyl-urea is introduced, it is apparently led by the methyl-urea group into the brain and causes tumours there. Previously the chemical causes for these particular tumours were completely unknown.

Nitrosamines are disintegrated very quickly by the body. Nevertheless insignificant doses of many of them are enough to cause cancer. High doses of them lead quickly to the death of the cells affected. The chief points of attack by nitrosamines seem to be the nucleic acids, the microsomes and various proteins in the cell plasma.

Other chemical carcinogens – lactones – also act as alkalysing agents. These compounds first began to interest cancer investigators when a group of scientists in the British chemical firm, ICI, induced sarcoma by injections of beta-propio-lactone. Eleven rats were inoculated subcutaneously with this compound; nine of them soon developed tumours in the neighbourhood of the injection sites.

Dangerous substances in nature

Cells can be damaged by substances other than those made in a laboratory. Among them is a long list of natural carcinogens. They include substances derived from the ripe berries of an asiatic mountain plant or from certain ground nuts formerly used in the United States and England to feed animals. A puzzling disease called "Turkey X" to which more than 100,000 turkeys succumbed in England in 1960, was traced indirectly, by the successful co-operation of laboratories in Europe and Africa, to a Brazilian groundnut on which these birds had been fed.

These ground nuts were infected with various strains of a very common fungus *Aspergillus flavus* which produces an antibiotic, aflatoxin. It first caused severe poisoning of the liver, and ultimately cancer developed. Aflatoxin has been found to be an extremely potent carcinogen in rats as well as in turkeys. Whereas in rats, for example, a daily dose of about 9,000 microgrammes of a potent chemical carcinogen is needed to cause tumours of the liver, 10 microgrammes of aflatoxin has the same effect. The chemical structure of aflatoxin has meanwhile been made known.

But some kinds of plants apparently also cause cancer in man. This assumption is mainly supported by observations which show that many groups of people with certain eating habits develop cancer more often than others. For example, cancer of the buccal cavity is found about 35 times more often in Ceylon, India and Singapore than in Europe.

Cancer epidemiologists ascribe this to the widespread habit of chewing betel in these areas. However, the betel nut itself seems not to be the carcinogenic factor; what these natives actually chew is areca nut wrapped in leaves of the plant *piper betel.*

Groundsel may also be carcinogenic. In many parts of Africa it is used for the preparation of tea or drugs. This could at least partly explain the astonishingly high incidence of primary cancer of the liver in Africa – in Europe tumours of the liver are almost exclusively derived from metastases from other organs.

Carcinogens in plants and foods

All these examples may be dismissed in Europe for the present as being both unusual and exotic. But the discovery that there are carcinogenic substances in widely distributed agricultural plants and popular foodstuffs in our latitudes will be depressing to many. But there is hardly any doubt, according to the most recent researches, that there are polycyclic hydrocarbons in salad, spinach, kale, grains and in many other vegetables and fruits.

At least eight aromatic hydrocarbons have, for example, been found in these natural foodstuffs by workers in the Hygiene-

Bacteriological Institute of Erlangen-Nuremberg as well as in the leaves of oak, beech, birch and other trees. Six of these aromatic hydrocarbons are certainly carcinogenic, among them the highly active 3, 4-benzpyrene.

In order to exclude chemical impurities, the experiments were carried out in regions far away from large housing estates or industrial areas. In some instances the plants were cultivated in a research station under protective plastic covers. But there still remained the possibility that carcinogens might enter the plants through their roots, from the soil.

In fact, carcinogens were also found in most humus soil. Dr. Walter Gräf, of the Erlangen Institute, assumes that these carcinogens have entered the soil through plants that have died. "The consequence of this," he wrote, "is that plants must be regarded as producers of carcinogenic, polycyclic, aromatic hydrocarbons."

The fact that these carcinogens are to be found in all plants suggested that they play an important part in plant metabolism, and further researches showed that benzpyrene dissolved in water causes a considerable acceleration of plant growth.

"It would be conceivable," wrote Dr. Gräf in the journal "Medizinische Klinik" "that these plant growth substances exert, by their action on animals and human cells, the function of a 'foreign hormone', which then brings about a plant-like, autonomous growth, i.e. a cancerous tumour." Benzpyrene was also found in human cells, such as lung tissues and bronchial lymphatic glands, but professional circles are generally agreed that this must be the result of substances introduced from outside. In animal cells, in contrast to plants there is apparently no benzpyrene at all.

Thus meat-eating would be less dangerous than vegetarianism. "Consequently," so Gräf says, "vegetarians would have to have a higher incidence of gastric cancer than meat eaters." The decline of gastric cancer in various countries could therefore be ascribed in part to the fact that mankind nowadays feeds chiefly on meat and other animal products. On the other hand it must be strongly emphasized that the amount of carcinogenic substances in plants is incredibly small, and can only be expressed in millionths of a gram per kilogram. Salad, according to the results hitherto obtained, contains the lowest content of benzpyrene; grains have the highest, especially after drying with certain mixtures of gas and air.

Divided views on arsenic

Long before benzpyrene became a recognised carcinogen, research workers concerned with vocational and environmental cancer were busy on metallic substances. An example of this was the small Silesian town of Reichenstein. For a thousand years, gold, silver and later arsenic ores were mined there. For a long time the drinking and ground water was contaminated with arsenic.

As a result of this – it seemed to the advocates of environmental cancer – many inhabitants of this region were afflicted by the most varied illnesses: liver diseases, skin diseases, digestive and nervous disturbances – and occasionally by malignant tumours. In some parts of Argentina and Formosa, where the water was contaminated by natural arsenic, cases of cancer were also observed. Whether they could be attributed to the arsenic was not proved.

On the other hand, Dr. William Hueper considers it certain that cancer can be caused by the consumption of wine made from grapes which have been treated with certain pesticides. Hueper worked, until his retirement, in the National Cancer Institute in Bethesda, and is an authority on environmental cancer. As he says; "Cancer can be caused in various human organs by modern pesticides. This demonstrates a general factor which is important in the causation of environmental cancer. Environmental factors can usually cause cancer in a variety of tissues, depending on the route by which the carcinogens enter the human body."

An incident in 1936 in Freiberg, Saxony, where there are silver and lead foundries, demonstrated that arsenic occasionally also constitutes a certain danger to animals. Arsenical fumes poured from these foundries into the air and settled on surrounding meadows, fields and orchards. Animals fed on plants from these subsequently showed numerous symptoms of disease, among which were malignant tumours.

Similarly, many investigators claim to have found cancerous diseases in human beings treated for a long time with arsenical preparations, previously used in the treatment of syphilis. The evidence for this is as scanty as the number of cases described. It is even more controversial whether arsenic actually causes cancer in animals. In the laboratory it has proved extremely difficult to induce skin or other forms of cancer in experimental animals. Therefore arsenic is probably only a very weak carcinogen.

Under certain conditions cancer can be caused in animals by metals. This was first reported in 1942 by Hans Rudolf Schinz in Zürich. He used small pieces of metal which he introduced into the thigh bones of rabbits. Since then there have been numerous publications on this subject, showing that various forms of cancer could be caused in animals by chromium, cobalt, nickel, selenium, lead and mercury.

Chrome, nickel and asbestos are also threatening causes of cancer in man, especially cancer of the respiratory organs. Both in the United States and Europe it has been shown that people who work with chromium show an unusally high incidence of cancer of the respiratory organs. Numerous experiments on animals have now been done on this. These show that sesquivalent chromium is apparently the most dangerous: trivalent or metallic chromium seems, on the other hand, not to be carcinogenic. Iron – the metal most used in modern engineering – has not yet been shown to be a cause of cancer in any of its forms.

How do metals cause cancer? To this question cancer investigators have at present little in the way of an answer. It is, however, assumed that it is the physical, rather than the chemical, characteristics of the metals that cause cancer, because most metals are inactive in the form of a powder. Sarcomas, or less frequently carcinomas, are only formed when the metals are put in the form of small discs or as metal foils into the bodies of experimental animals. Perhaps these metals exert a disturbing influence on the enzyme systems, the regulators of cell growth.

Bakelite discs in the tissues

Plastics may also cause cancer in animals – but only if a certain experimental finesse is used. In 1942 the American surgeon F. C. Turner implanted small bakelite discs, which were surrounded by a carcinogenic hydrocarbon, under the skin of a rat. When he removed these plates some time later, there were no tumours. Turner then repeated this experiment with similar plates without the carcinogenic covering. He found that if the plates were present for long enough in the tissues, sarcomas developed.

Six years later the American couple B. S. and Enid Oppenheimer came upon an astonishing fact. They found that sarcomas had formed in rats whose kidneys, when young, had been wrapped in cellophane film. This was intended to induce a high blood pressure. In this case the latent period of development of cancer was just over a year. Further experiments again produced tumours and these were identified as sarcomas by further transplantations. Ultimately the German investigator Hans. U. Zollinger also reported similar results independently of the Oppenheimers. The result was that plastic films and plates became a focus of interest in experimental research on cancer. Sarcomas were caused in animals by polyethylene, polyvinylchloride, and many other plastics used in the household – and also by nylon and polyester threads. But the work of Dr. Hans Nothdurft of Heidelberg showed that the causation of tumours depends not so much on the synthetic material itself as on the form and size of the material used.

Here also, as with metals, scientists interpret the carcinogenic effect more by physical than chemical processes. All these substances consist of macromolecules in which thousands of individual atom groups join together in chains to form a giant molecule. Perhaps the carcinogenic effect can be due to this characteristic of the molecule. "The present experimental results" says David B. Clayson of the Cancer Research Institute of the University of Leeds "do not, however, permit a reasonable estimate of the potential dangers of these substances."

Do we live in an "Ocean of Carcinogens"?

The list of suspected substances could be enlarged still further. As has already been mentioned, the World Health Organisation has recorded about 450 such substances and their number is increasing.

Does mankind therefore actually live in an "Ocean of Carcinogens", as many people, since Rachel Carson's much discussed best-seller "The Silent Spring" have feared? Is cancer the price of the progress of civilisation, the punishment for mankind's interference with its natural environment, as philosophers weary of civilisation have thought?

Even cancer investigators are divided on these questions. K. H. Bauer in Heidelberg expects a considerable reduction of cancerous disease from a "sanitary revolution", a complete ban on all

The whole of cancer research concentrates on the differences between normal and malignant cells. These differences may appear in all parts of the cell, as for example in our electronmicroscope photograph, in the nucleus.

1. Healthy plasma
2. Viruses
3. Vacuoles
4. Healthy nucleus
5. Nuclear membrane
6. Cell membrane
7. A mitochondrion
8. An altered nucleus

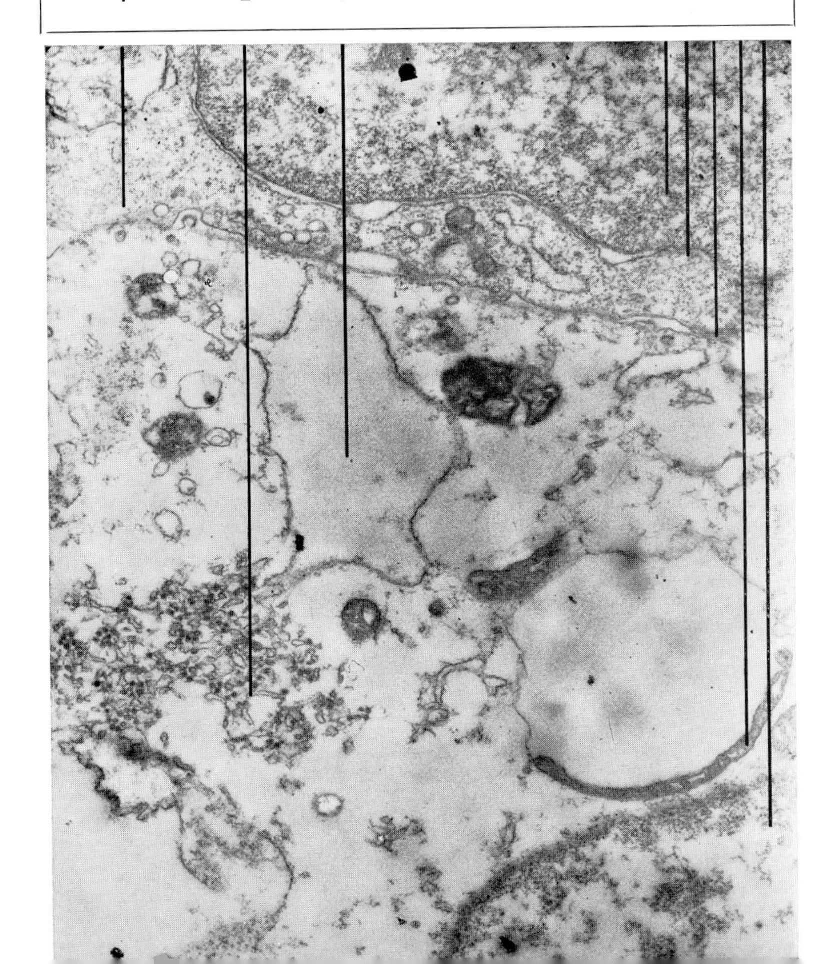

Diagram and an electron microscope photograph of a normal cell.

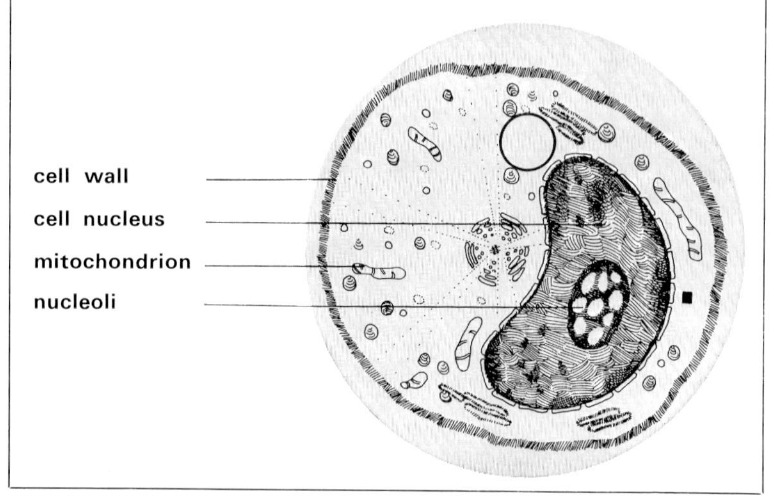

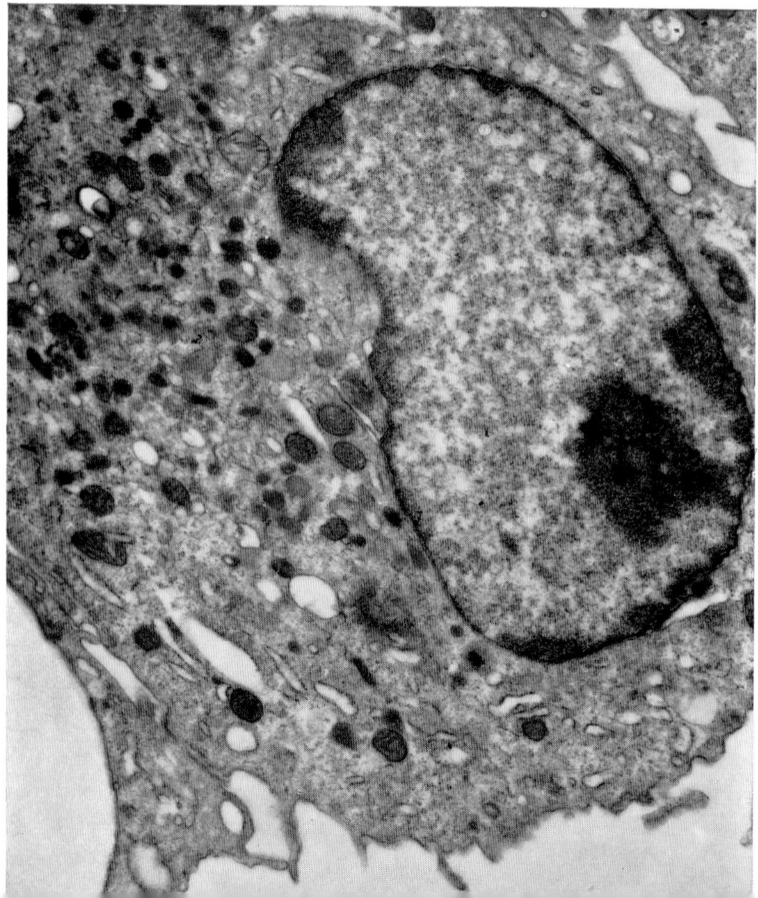

Diagram of the formation of a tumour in normal tissue, from the first malignant cell to a tumour that can be clinically diagnosed. The photograph shows a thin section of a fully-developed tumour.

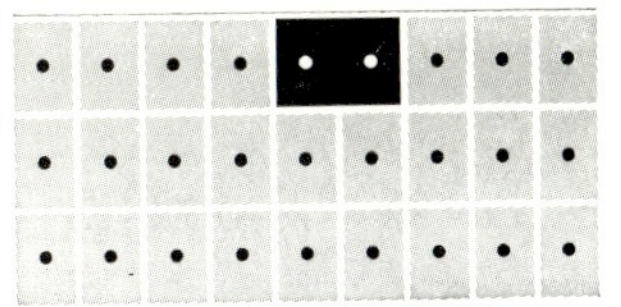

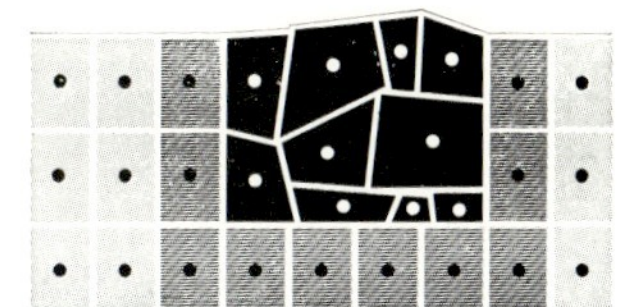

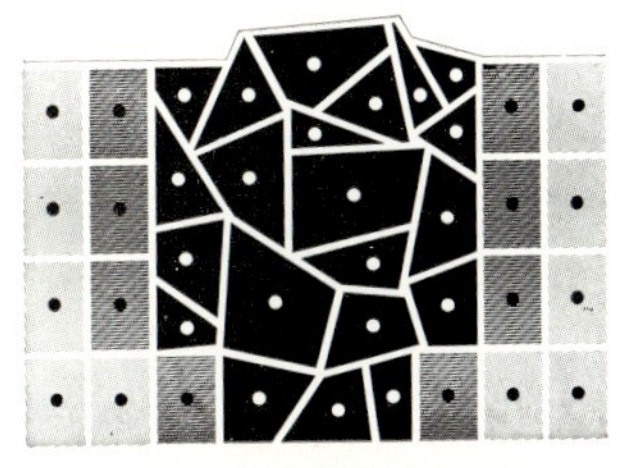

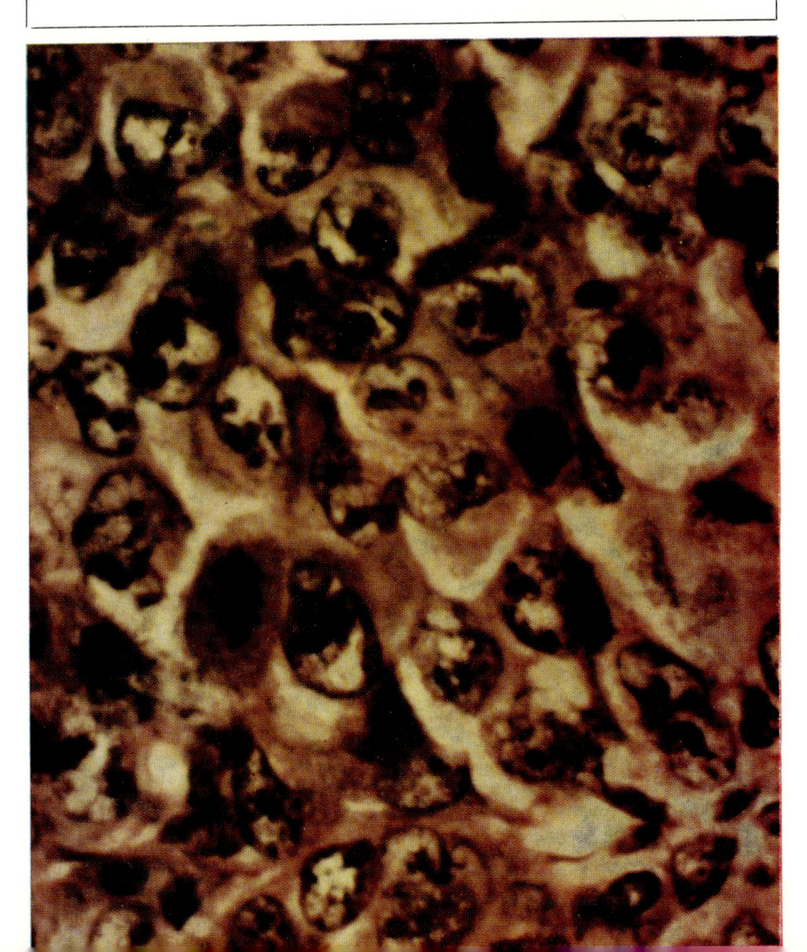

Rudolf Virchow (top) the founder of cell pathology. Paul Ehrlich (bottom) the creator of chemotherapy.
The mouse carcinoma shown in the coloured photograph bears his name. Since 1906 it has been transmitted through innumerable phases to animals all over the world.

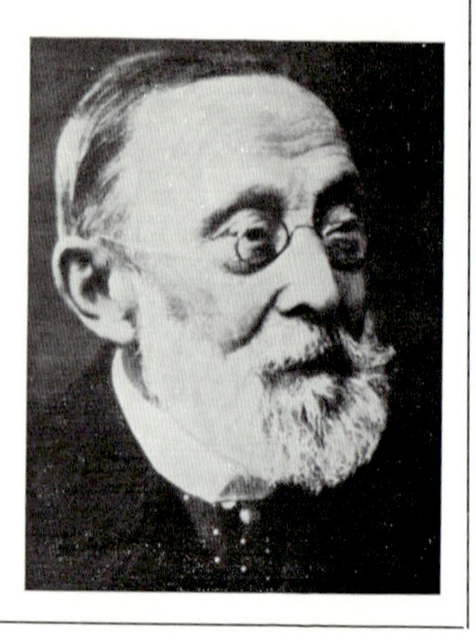

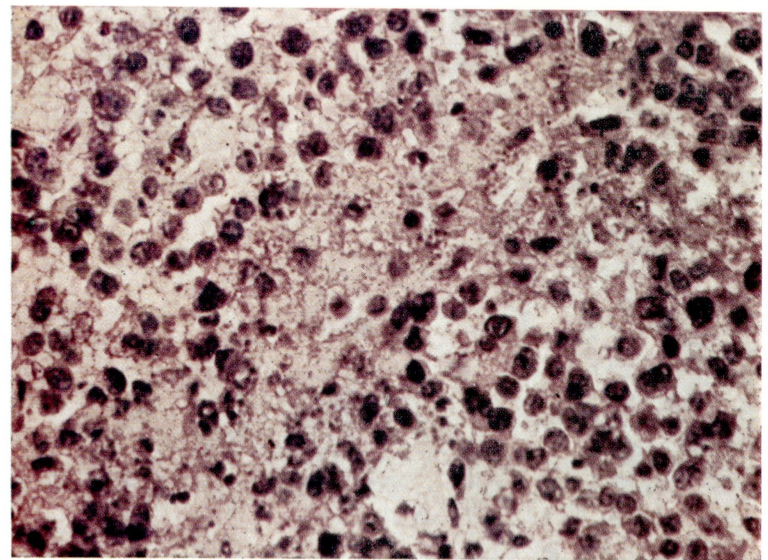

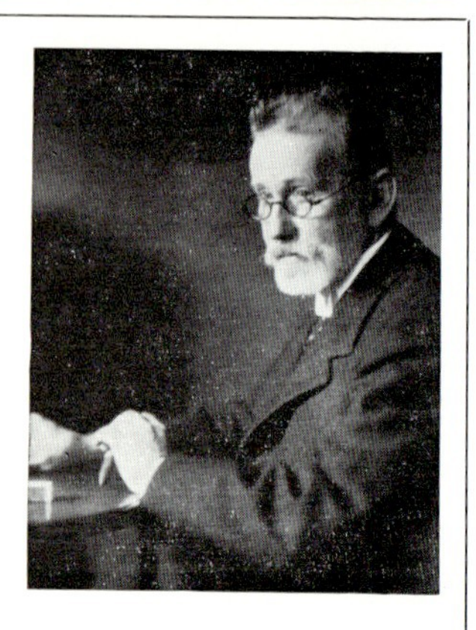

Isolated cells can be multiplied and cultivated further in tissue culture, which is an important aid to the study of metabolism and of the morphology and genetic changes in the cells. The microphotograph shows such a culture.

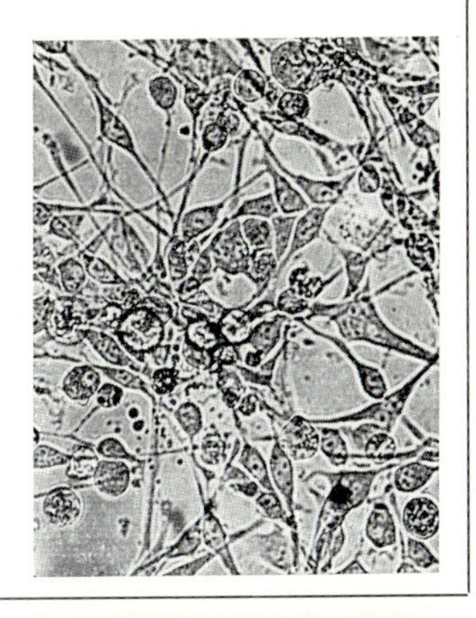

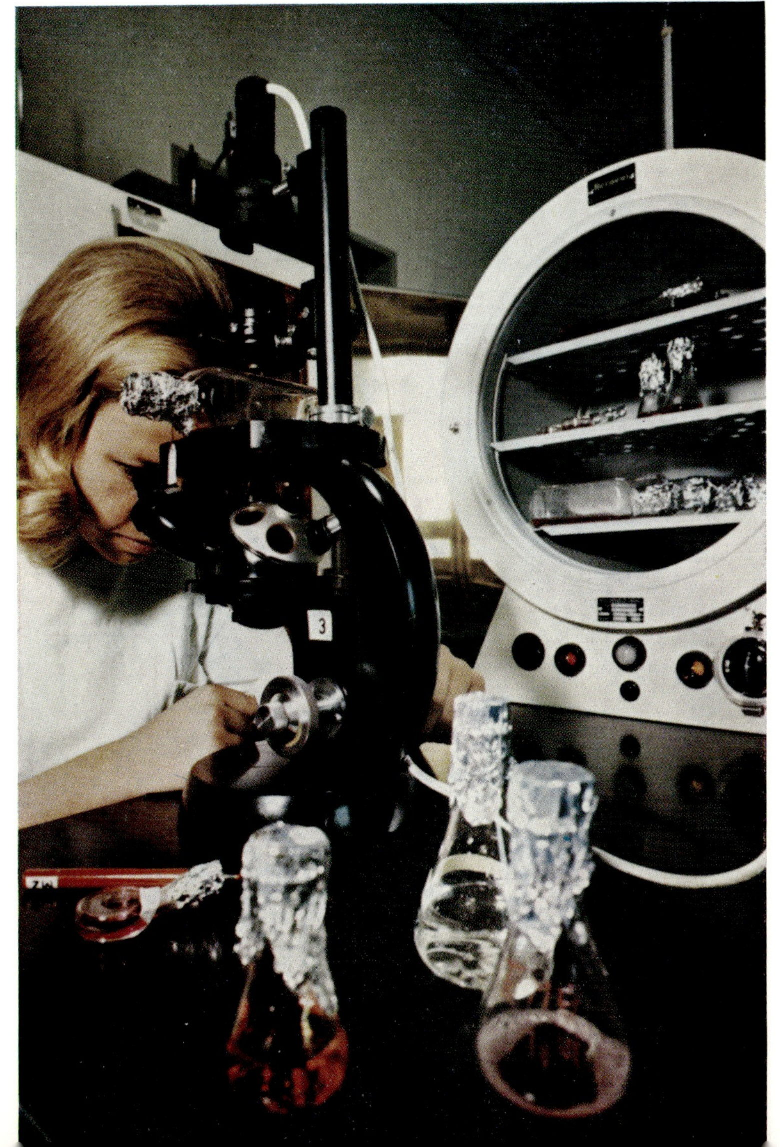

The quartet of research workers (from left to right) Miescher, Avery, Crick and Watson, who have, during the last hundred years, made important contributions to the study of nucleic acids.

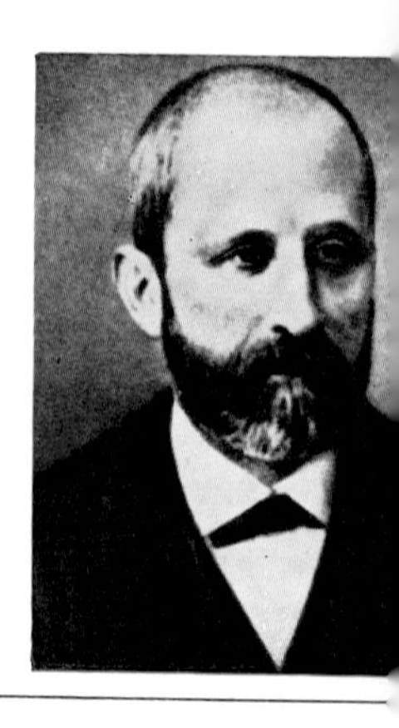

The two models show different ways of illustrating the structure of DNA molecules. They show the two interwoven strands composed of phosphorus and sugar groups. Between them are the "Rungs" composed of the two pairs of bases.

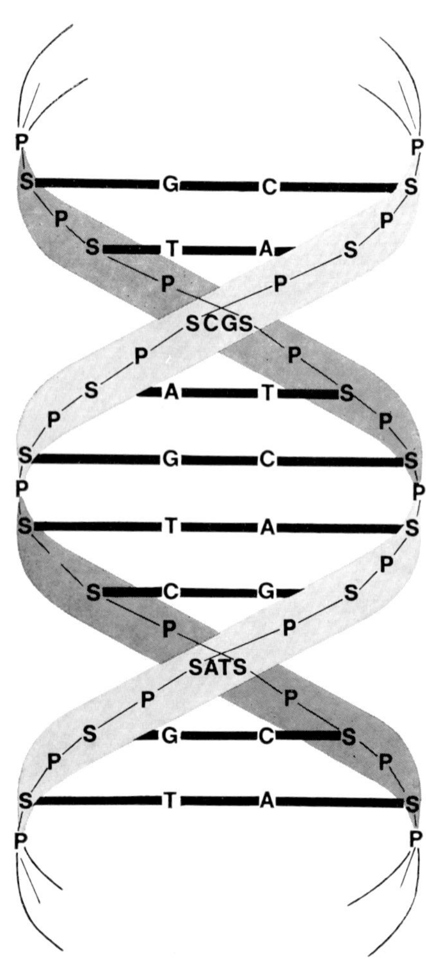

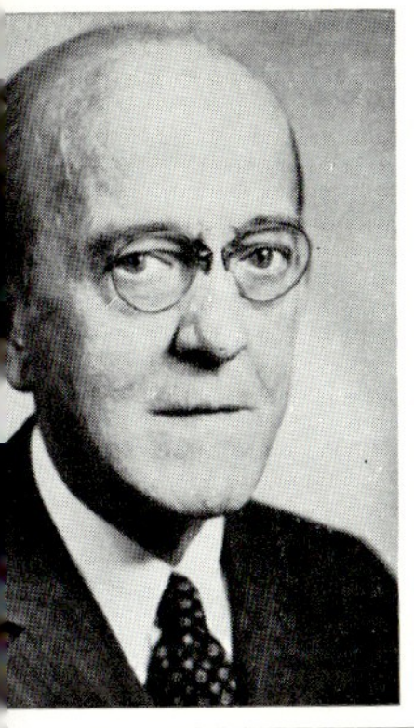

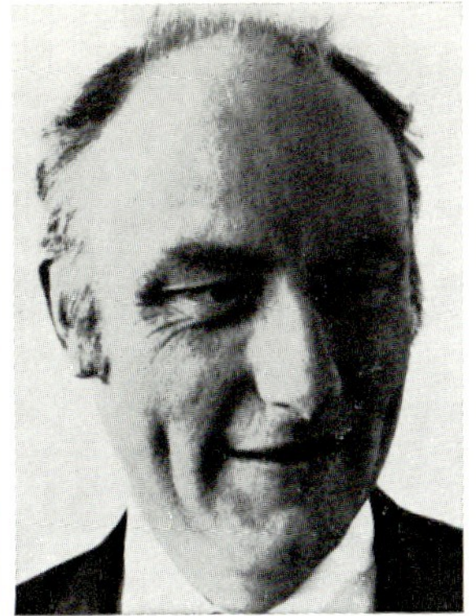

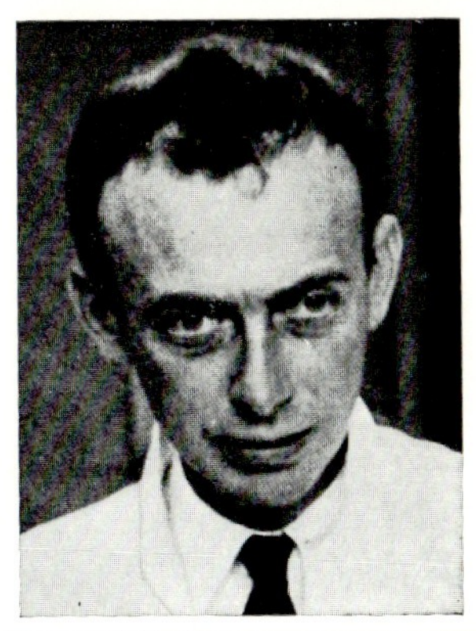

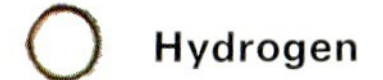

Hydrogen

Oxygen

Carbon

Phosphorus

Thymine

Adenine

Guanine

Cytosine

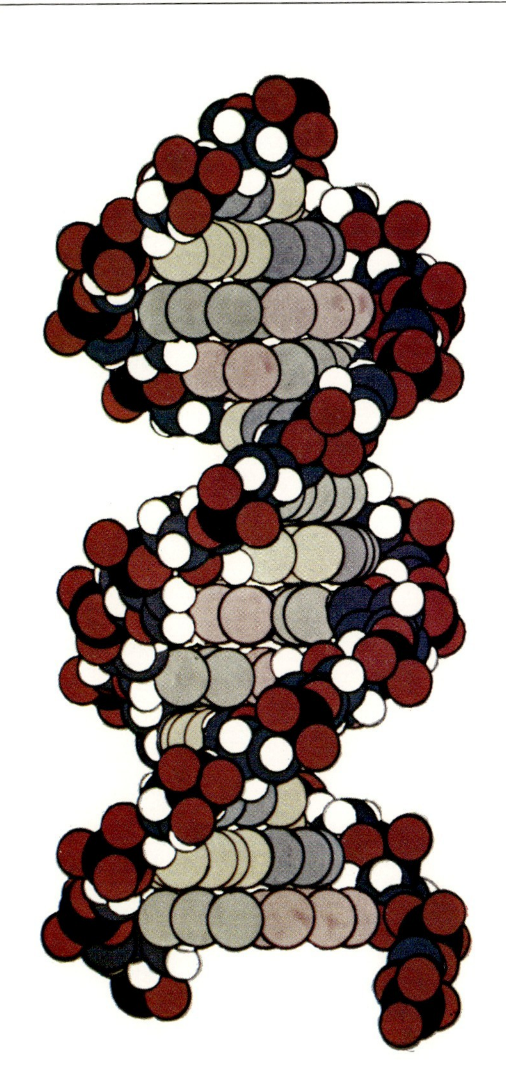

Chromosomes carry the hereditary characters; schematic arrangements facilitate comparative studies.

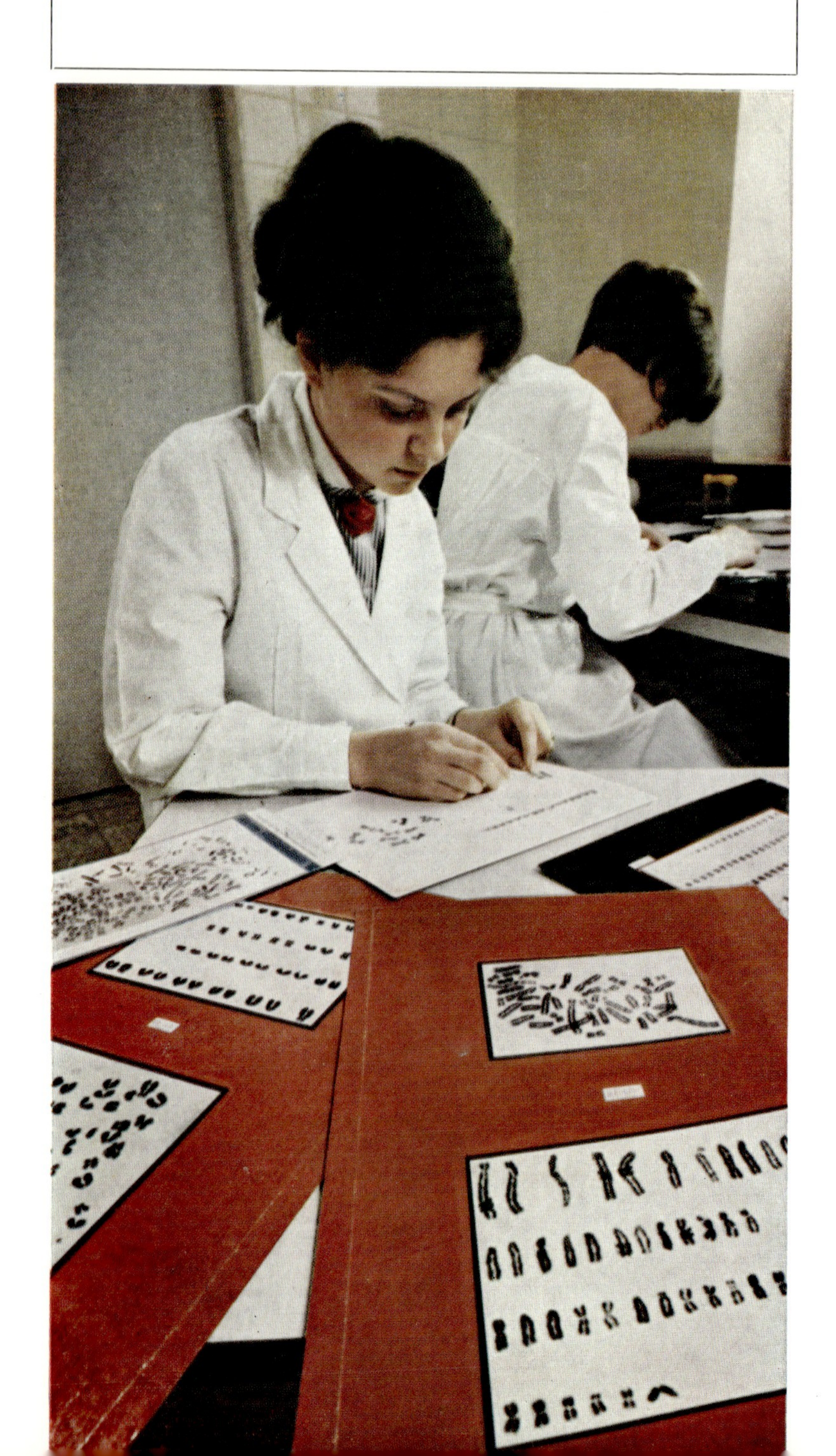

suspected poisons. No less experienced scientists, on the other hand, refer to statistics which show that, out of 4 million cases of cancer between 1900 and 1950, only 500 were caused by chemicals. Professor Heinz Oettel, of the Badische Anilin-und-Sodafabrik, writes that: "External chemical influences cannot – except for cigarette smoking – have anything like the significance ascribed to them as causes of human cancer."

A sober view shows, in fact, that the only thing we know with certainty about most carcinogenic substances is that they cause cancer in animals. But many substances that are very carcinogenic in experiments on animals have only an extremely weak effect on man, (like tar), or no effect at all, (like gold). Conversely, compounds such as chromates, which can cause tumours in man when administered for a long time, are not carcinogenic in experiments on animals. But even with carcinogenic substances the causation of cancer only succeeds in certain animals and in certain sites of application, and with the aid of extremely high doses under conditions to which there is little chance that man will be exposed.

The former Director of the Experimental Pathology division of the Farbenfabriken Bayer, Dr. Christian Hackmann therefore said, "One can, by analogy to the observations made on experimental animals, suppose that exogenous poisons also play a part in man. But in most cases definite connections with certain pathogenic agents cannot clearly be determined."

Thus, Hackmann says, it has still not been established in a scientifically convincing manner whether carcinogenic substances in human foods can be blamed for the very common cancer of the digestive organs. "Even if we assume that carcinogenic factors in food have significance, we can say nothing about what kind of factors these are. Only in vocational cancer can the relationship between the pathogenic agents and the origin of tumours be investigated and more or less clearly detected. Occupational cancers, however, comprise only a small portion and play a less important part in the total picture of human cancers."

Occupational cancers constitute roughly only one per cent of all kinds of cancer. Among approximately 500 cases of vocational cancer in Germany which Professor Oettel mentioned during the first 50 years of this century, 350 were cases of cancer of the bladder, 90 were cancer due to chromates and 10 each were due to arsenic, asbestos and tar.

Causes often remain hidden

For many people suffering from cancer, the initial cause of their disease cannot be identified with complete certainty, nor can the effect of one or more carcinogens be determined. This is mainly due to the characteristic latent period, which can last for decades. In animals this latent period often lasts only a few weeks or months. "And a criminal" thinks the Münster specialist Professor Werner H. Hauss, "who is not caught red-handed, usually escapes human justice".

Dr. Frank L. Horsfall, President of the Sloan-Kettering Institute, also attributes to the chemical causes of cancer a quite limited effect. "The number of chemical compounds," he thinks, "which are definitely recognised as inducing cancer in man, is not large. They seem to act chiefly on epithelial structures and, among these, especially on the skin, the bladder and respiratory tract. Pitch, tar and oils are presumably the main culprits in skin cancer in industry."

Horsfall holds it as still incompletely established that the hydrocarbons in these substances are responsible for cancer. Among the five or more compounds which may contribute to cancer of the bladder are, as has been said, beta-napthylamine, and benzidine. Chromium, various metal compounds and asbestos are the chief factors which have been related to cancer of the human respiratory tract, especially of the lungs. As is well-known, man must be exposed to these industrial products for a very long time, usually for years or even decades, and "only then does cancer develop and its incidence does not seem to be very high".

The chemical origins of cancer: an unsolved problem

The part played by chemicals as causes of cancer seems to Dr. Frank L. Horsfall to be at present "more a matter for speculation and debate than an established fact". The field of the chemical origin of cancer is still full of unsolved problems. "Our present experimental methods are inadequate and insufficiently convincing to assess the significance of environmental factors in relation to the appearance of malignant tumours." Horsfall refers to yet another interesting fact: though it is undisputed that numerous chemical compounds may cause cancer in certain experimental animals, there is so far no proof that human cells in tissue culture can be caused to become malignant by the direct effect of such compounds.

Dr. David B. Clayson, of the Cancer Research Institute of the University of Leeds in England, takes the view, however, that we must depend primarily on animal experiments in investigating possible chemical causes of cancer. But why should man react to carcinogens in a completely different way from animals? Dr. John Weisburger, of the National Cancer Institute, who together with his wife Elizabeth is considered to be one of the most successful investigators of cancer in the U.S.A., is of the opinion that: "A chemical compound which, according to the evidence, causes cancer in one or two kinds of animals, will very probably do this in other kinds and may well do so also in man." Clayson admits that at present we cannot demonstrate precisely how man reacts to chemical carcinogens. "We do not therefore know exactly to what extent it is necessary to protect the human population against carcinogens which have been proved to be carcinogenic in animals."

Thus the relationship between chemical substances and cancer gives rise today to two widely divergent views. Some scientists would ban every chemical compound that has caused a tumour in some animals. Others consider that such a demand – for the time being at least – is much too sweeping. The results of experiments on animals, they say, have little or no significance for human cancer. Clayson takes a middle position: "At present every compound that has caused a large number of tumours in experiments on animals, should be considered as dangerous also to man. Precautionary measures must be taken in every instance, and men should be saved from contact with such substances either in their work or environment."

The two-stage theory

Varied as are the chemical causes of cancer, so for the most part are their modes of action and potency. Some chemical substances are very weak carcinogens – they cause cancer only in association with other substances – the chief carcinogen thus being combined with another. This theory of co-carcinogenesis was established by experiments carried out more than 20 years ago in Oxford by I. Berenblum and Philip Shubik. Today Berenblum works in the Weizmann Institute in Israel and Shubik in the Chicago Medical School.

When Berenblum and Shubik painted mice only once with a very potent carcinogenic hydrocarbon – benzpyrene or 7, 12 dimethylbenzanthracene – no cancer resulted. But when the same parts of the skin of these mice were later painted with croton oil, which itself has no carcinogenic effect, the animals promptly developed first papillomata and then tumours.

This suggests that the hydrocarbon had made the cells malignant, but that their transformation had remained unrecognisable. The biological completion of the process required a further step. Or to put it in concrete form: the first compound started the malignant process, but the cells remained latent. A tumour was formed only under the influence of a new factor.

From these observations developed an interesting and much-discussed hypothesis, which was briefly touched upon in Chapter 1. According to it there must be, in cancer caused by chemical substances, two or even three definite stages. Stage 1 is caused by the "initiating factor", Stage 2, by the "promoting factor", whilst Stage 3 is the formation of the tumour. One of the "initiating factors" most often used in experiments is urethane, which is chiefly used as a narcotic for animals. The classical "promoting agent" is still croton oil. This is not a chemically pure substance, but a mixture of compounds that can only be defined with difficulty.

Professor Erich Hecker, of the German Cancer Research Centre in Heidelberg, has succeeded in elucidating at least some of the active principles in croton oil, and now that some of its constituents have been synthesized, sufficient quantities of a "pure", chemically well-defined substance are available for further experiments on animals. Croton oil has so far proved to be "co-carcinogenic" only on the skin of mice. In rats, rabbits or hamsters it fails as a second factor in the chemical origin of cancer.

Hormones: agents or accomplices?

We cannot yet say whether there is such a two- or three-stage mechanism in the formation of tumours in man. Professor Oettel writes: "Probably in human cancer the combined action of different factors – co-carcinogenesis – plays a greater part than has been so far detected." The rather complex word "syncarcinogenesis", coined by Professor Bauer, embodies the idea that different carcinogenic stimuli act on the cells of a tissue either simultaneously or successively. In this way not just a summation of their effects could occur but a potentiation. A tumour would be, in this view, the combined result of many carcinogenic influences and of an effect of favourable internal influences, such as a certain liability to cancer.

There is today little doubt that various hormones are included in these "internal influences". More disputed are the questions whether hormones merely exert a favourable influence in cancer; whether they are only accessories, or can also independently start the cancer process. It is supposed that a relationship between malignant growth and the effects of hormones could exist in two particular forms of cancer: in cancer of the breast – the most common cancer in women – and in cancer of the prostate gland in men.

In 1896 a surgeon in Glasgow was able to report to his colleagues a sensational event. Sir Thomas Beatson had arrested for some time the progress of an advanced cancer of the breast in a young woman by removing her ovaries.

At that time even the greatest scientific authorities knew less about hormones than is taught today to intelligent schoolboys. As is now well-known, hormones are formed in endocrine glands and are discharged directly into the bloodstream. From this they often pass into far distant organs and there operate in minimal dosages.

In recent decades, knowledge of the endocrine glands has developed in a striking manner. For some time there has been no doubt that hormones play a decisive part in the chemical processes of the cell. They promote or inhibit the growth of the organism, direct the utilisation of sugars and their conversion into energy; they control the excretion of water, reproduction, and hundreds of other important functions of life. It has been truly said that hormones decide between dwarfs and giants.

Central control by the hypophysis

The hypophysis (pituitary gland) functions like the conductor in the endocrine orchestra of the body. It is situated in the brain, but weighs less than a gram. It is divided into an anterior and a posterior lobe, and it largely controls the secretions of the other endocrine glands. The sexual glands, the adrenals and the thyroid are dependent to a high degree on this tiny cerebral appendage. In addition, the hypophysis produces somatropin in its anterior lobe, and vasopressin and oxytocin in its posterior lobe. Many endocrinologists assume, however, that the hypophysis is not completely autonomous. It is apparently dependent to some degree on the hypothalamus in the mid-brain, and on the endocrine glands in the various organs of the body. These glands can, by a kind of "feedback", exert certain influences on the control centre, the hypophysis. This complicated system of effects and counter-effects can therefore be compared to the mode of action of a thermostat.

But it is always the hypophysis which gives the first impulse for the rest of the hormone production in the body. For example, the formation of the hormones of the female sex glands proceeds as follows: the hypophysis produces in its anterior lobe two sex hormones, namely prolan A and B. These hormones pass by way of the blood to the ovaries, where, under the influence of prolan A, a Graafian follicle bursts and the egg thus set free passes through the oviduct into the uterus. The prolan B. on the other hand, starts, in the now egg-free follicle, the production of another hormone, the corpus luteum hormone, (progesterone).

Together with the follicle hormone (oestrogen) this corpus luteum hormone acts on the mucosa of the uterus and causes an enlargement of the cells in this organ. In short, it prepares completely for the establishment of the fertilised egg in the uterus.

Follicle hormones and corpus luteum hormones concentrate their action more or less exclusively on the female sex organs. But they also influence the skin, bone-marrow and many processes in cells and tissues.

What happens when, under the influence of the hypophysis, too much or too little of the hormones are produced in the tissues dependent on them? In that case, a whole series of serious disease symptoms can develop. In general it can be said: if not enough growth hormone is produced, the dependent tissues develop too feebly. An excess of hormones, on the other hand leads to their excessive development.

At this point the study of hormones leads to the study of cancer. If certain hormones should cause growth that is too vigorous, can this not lead under certain conditions to cancer? Is it only by chance that cancer in the female body chooses most frequently the two organs which are constantly under the influence of the sex hormones? For at least thirty years the female breast and uterus are exposed every month to an "alternating bath" of hormones. And it is precisely these organs which are most often affected by cancer.

When the hormones fail

Many scientists ascribe a more important place in the mosaic of human cancer to the hormones than to any other chemical substances. Hormones are always present in the body of every human being. On the other hand only a small portion of the population is exposed to chemical substances. Scientists must, however, rely for their study of the relationships between cancer and hormones to a great extent upon experiments on animals. The first such experiments on a large scale were done in 1916. The American cancer investigator Leo Loeb and his colleague A. E. C. Lathrop of the Washington University School of Medicine, St. Louis, removed the ovaries from young mice. The mice belonged to a strain in which spontaneous breast cancer is very common. But after this operation not one animal developed this disease. On the other hand, young male mice developed malignant tumours when female ovaries were implanted in them. Normally these male mice did not develop breast cancer.

These initial experiments were followed by a large number of others, in which either additional hormones were given to animals or the supply of certain hormones was cut off, so causing cancer. When synthetic sex hormones became available, it also became possible to administer exactly measured doses.

The French cancer investigator Antoine Lacassagne injected mouse follicle hormone subcutaneously and was able in this way to increase the frequency of breast cancer. He was even able to use oestrogens to cause breast cancer in male animals. If animals were given very high doses of oestrogen for a long time, tumours developed in the uterus, testes, liver, kidneys and bladder, and leukaemia also developed. Dr. William U. Gardner of Yale University in America was one of the first to trace all these forms of cancer to a disturbance in hormone balance. He also succeeded in causing tumours in the endocrine glands: tumours of the hypophysis, thyroid, sexual and adrenal glands.

Disturbances of the hormone equilibrium occur if co-operation ceases between the hypophysis in the brain and one of the local glands. As has already been indicated, there is a very labile regulation system between the hypophysis and the local glands. In this way the production of hormones in the sex glands or the thyroid is regulated and adjusted to the right amount. As soon as the hormone level needed has been reached and sufficient secretion has been discharged, this is recorded in the hypophysis by feedback. The production of the organotropic agent is stopped. When the local hormone production falls below the required level, the hypophysis switches itself on again in order to hold the production at exactly the right level.

However, one of the glands in this automatic system may fail. It gives out too little or even no secretion. Then the hypophysis will unfailingly produce more organotropic hormone and send it to this gland. If the hypophysis is forced in this way into overproduction, cancer may ultimately result. Under certain conditions the hypophysis itself is thus affected; otherwise it will be the local gland which has been constantly stimulated to excessive hormone production. Collapse of hormone balance can be artificially induced by removal of the local glands by operation, by irradiation or by chemicals. Because the secretion of the glands is then absent, the hypophysis will continuously send out excessive quantities of organotropic hormone. The malignant process is started.

Other tumours may also be caused by the "chief gland". If, for example, the sexual glands are removed from animals, the hypophysis may produce unlimited quantities of the hormone which should control them. The result is that either the hypophysis itself is affected, or malignant tumours develop in the adrenal cortex. Sex hormones are formed not only in the sex glands, but also – in smaller quantities – by the adrenal cortex. If the sex glands are absent the hypophysis concentrates the whole of its production on the cortex, in order to restore the hormone balance.

Tumours of the ovary can also be induced in mice and rats if their ovaries are implanted into the spleen. Even in this situation these glands produce the corresponding hormone, but since it passes into the liver and is inactivated there, it is lacking in the blood circulation. Consequently the hypophysis continues to produce its gonadotropic hormone, and overproduction may ultimately result in malignant tumours.

The list of such experiments on animals could be extended in many directions, for there is hardly any kind of tumour which man cannot produce in animals with the use of hormones. It has been possible to obtain results that are in themselves highly interesting, but from whicvh no conclusions can be drawn that are generally applicable to human cancer. For this reason it is still not known whether hormones play a predominant or only a secondary rôle in human cancer. Possibly they only prepare the way, by increasing cell activity, for the action of "complete carcinogens", as is shown perhaps by most of the chemical causes of cancer.

Faulty synthesis in the body

Whether or not hormones are to be regarded as "incomplete carcinogens" and the polycyclic hydrocarbons as "complete" ones, there is an amazing similarity between these two classes of substance. The hormones of the adrenal cortex and the sex glands belong to the chemical group of steroids, and the carcinogenic hydrocarbons differ little from that group. This fact has set cancer investigators thinking for a long time past. Could it not be, many of them ask themselves, that the organism from time to time undergoes a faulty synthesis – nothing short of suicidal – by which certain hormone steroids are changed into carcinogenic hydrocarbons?

The following would be conceivable: during the replication of the sex hormones there are mistakes. The resulting errors in the biochemical process lead to the formation of substances which are carcinogenic. If this process lasts long enough, if the organism does not correct the faulty production in time, tumour cells may be formed. Every clinician sees innumerable cases of cancer for which it is impossible to find the slightest explanation. They could be ascribed, if the foregoing theory is correct, to a fault in the patient's own body.

At present there is no proof of such a theory that cancer can arise "from within" – at any rate, in man. But should it not at least be possible in the laboratory to change steroids into carcinogenic hydrocarbons? In fact, the German scientist Heinrich Wieland, Professor of Chemistry in Munich and Nobel Laureate for 1927, succeeded in doing this. He changed one of the best-known steroids, a bile acid, through a series of chemical intermediate stages into 20-methylcholanthrene, one of the most potent carcinogens known today. Methylcholanthrene leads, for example, to breast cancer in mice and rats. This occurs if it is painted on the relevant parts of the skin, given by the mouth, or implanted in the form of tiny pellets into the breast tissue.

Usually these tumours can only develop with favourable hormonal conditions. It has been discovered that the carcinogens methylcholanthrene and dibenzanthracene also have a certain hormonal effect. Dibenzanthracene has oestrogenic properties. It promotes, for example, the growth of certain parts of the breast. Methylcholanthrene, like progesterone, promotes uterine development. Hitherto, admittedly, it has been possible to change bile acids into carcinogenic methylcholanthrene only in the test tube, and many cancer investigators therefore doubt that such a metamorphosis is possible in a living organism. They point out that biochemical carcinogens have never been found in the urine or liver of people suffering from cancer. On the other hand, biochemists emphasize the fact that each of the chemical steps in the change from bile acids into methylcholanthrene could be accomplished with the help of known enzyme reactions. Why should the organism not be capable of these processes, if it accomplishes more difficult chemical transformations than those that can be achieved by any laboratory in the world? The suspicion that cancers of metabolic organs, such as the liver or pancreas, arise through metabolic products in the body itself, can at present be only vaguely established. Nevertheless, cancer research cannot afford to ignore such assumptions; it must follow them up by every possible scientific means.

Yet another trail deserves attention. This involves one of the amino acids necessary for protein synthesis. It has been discovered that, in one of these essential amino acids – tryptophane – metabolic faults may occur which convert it into a cause of cancer of the bladder. The hide-bound view of many investigators that cancer may be exclusively conditioned by environment, and caused by certain external agents, is thus continually threatened.

Psychic influences as unknown factors

Psychic and emotional factors may also play a part in the cancerous process. This does not mean that even extraordinary psychic stresses can change healthy cells into malignant ones. However, certain stress situations may perhaps stimulate already present tumour cells to greater activity and increased growth, or may negatively influence the body's defence against such cells. American cancer investigators are anxious not to exclude this possibility.

Several investigators presented instructive reports on this subject to a meeting of the New York Academy of Science in 1965. Dr. Arthur Schmale, Jnr., of the University of Rochester, considered the possibility that heavy emotional blows, such as the death of a near relative, could be an important factor in the development of cancer. The particular kind of despair shown by women affected by such events, has led Schmale in many cases to the diagnosis of cancer. Subsequent clinical investigations had verified this.

This report clearly contradicts another group of American doctors who had examined women for breast cancer. Each woman was carefully asked, before the physical examination, whether she had suffered a painful separation for some time from her mother, father or some other person she loved. No relationship could be found between events of this kind and greater frequency of breast cancer.

An English doctor reported to the same Congress of the New York Academy of Science his experiences with patients with lung cancer. Many of these people found it difficult to relieve their pent-up feelings. Dr. David Kissen, of the Southern General Hospital in Glasgow, inclined therefore to the opinion that excessive mental stress can considerably increase the risk of cancer that arises from cigarette smoking.

There are even observations on animals relating to the problem of cancer and the emotions. Scientists in the National Cancer Institute in the United States have, for example, discovered that mice kept alone in a cage developed cancer of the breast earlier and more often than mice kept together. Also, animals subjected to shocks, such as heat or surgical operations, were appreciably more vulnerable to cancer.

Psychic stresses of this kind undoubtedly affect the internal secretory glands and the hormone level. In particular, adrenalin produced by the adrenal cortex is excreted in appreciably greater quantities in cases of physical or psychic stress. For this reason the adrenal hormone has been called the "stress hormone". But the thyroid and the sex glands are also sensitive to psychic stress.

It cannot be proved that the increased production of hormones caused by such psychic factors may lead, in the long run, to cancer. Many investigators consider that just the reverse is possible; that a hormone system that is in a state of chronic malfunction leads, in the course of time, to cancer and through this to psychic disturbances. In general, however, the relationship between psychic influences and cancer is not widely investigated, and at present not even a working hypothesis is possible.

Cancer from radiation: an intensive study

Although there are still many questions relating to cancer caused by chemical substances or hormones, scientists are on much surer ground when it comes to cancer caused by radiation. There has been no doubt for many decades, for example, that Röntgen rays, which reveal so many diseases and help to cure them, have in return taken a cruel toll in many cases.

The luminous dial industry in the American State of New Jersey, which flourished particularly in the 1920's, is an example that is often quoted. This was a branch of industry that was still very young. The Frenchman Henri Bequerel, had first shown in 1896 that certain uranium salts emit rays that are very similar to X-rays discovered a year earlier by Röntgen. Two years later, the same phenomena were found by Marie Curie and her husband Pierre in thorium salts and pitch blende, ultimately they hit upon the name "radioactive" to describe substances of this kind.

Radioactivity can be traced to various elements, of which a whole series was subsequently discovered, among them radium, thorium, polonium, uranium and others. The atoms of such elements disintegrate without any external cause, and during this disintegration high energy radiation is set free. This consists partly of pieces of the disintegrated atoms, and partly of very short wave-radiations that are similar to Röntgen rays.

When zinc blende is struck by the high energy particles it emits light; from this discovery the idea of applying a mixture of radioactive material and zinc blende to the hands and dials of clocks, so that they could be seen in the dark, naturally followed. In the luminous dial industry of the United States hundreds of women were employed to put the radioactive mixture on the hands and dials of wrist watches. They used the finest brushes; in order that the brush should remain pointed enough for this accurate work, the women used the simplest and most effective method. They drew the brush from time to time between their lips.

After some years these women workers suddenly began to show curious symptoms of disease: purulent inflammations of the sockets of the teeth which did not heal. These were followed by such severe affections of the jaw bones and gums that some patients died of them. Cancer awaited the survivors. In 1928 the first bone sarcoma was found, and in 1931 nine cases were known. Ultimately this number increased to a total of 42. It was certain that the careless handling of the radioactive substance was the cause of these cancers.

It had been known for a long time that Röntgen rays and radioactive rays could cause cancer. When the rays were discovered in 1895, scientists were completely ignorant of their dangers. But over-enthusiastic and careless association with the new rays soon provided the bitter experience that the human body can be much harmed by strong and frequent Röntgen irradiation. The first effects of this radiation were burns on the skin, X-ray dermatitis; these were followed by chronic ulcers which resisted any treatment and would not heal. The third stage was cancer.

The first "X-ray cancer" was described in 1902. The victim of it was an employee in an X-ray tube factory, whose hand had constantly been used for photographic tests. A cancerous tumour developed on the back of the hand which made it necessary to amputate the arm. The discoverer of radioactive irradiation, Henri Bequerel, also experienced its dangers. Carelessly, he once put radium, which he wished to show during a lecture in London, into his waistcoat pocket for the journey, and as a result suffered severe burns.

Scientists cannot at present give a complete and satisfactory explanation of how radioactive and X-rays cause cancer. However, hypotheses have been developed which are highly probable. Because a malignant tumour only arises when cancer cells divide and transmit their malignant properties to daughter cells, the point of attack by the rays seems clear. The attack must be on the hereditary substance, and therefore on the DNA or RNA. After the irradiation of cells, important changes in the chromosomes have, in fact, been found. The chromosomes become sticky, and in division are no longer able to separate cleanly from one another – they remain linked in certain places or get into wrong positions. They may also be cut or broken, and then fail to re-join correctly.

It has been found that mutations occur under irradiation 150 times more often than under normal conditions. Moreover, in irradiation of RNA and DNA chemical changes are caused by which the DNA loses the ability to form certain enzymes. These effects are partly the result of direct hits by the rays on the DNA molecules. But they may also be indirect, namely via the formation of free radicals in the cell fluid.

Other forms of damage are conceivable. Rays not only hit the cell nucleus, but also the cytoplasm or the mitochondria, the significance of which has still not yet been fully established. Furthermore, the cell membrane, through which the important metabolic exchange of the cell occurs, becomes considerably more permeable under radiation. A series of changes in the cell metabolism may result from this. Irradiated cells also become much more susceptible to infections, especially to viruses. If viruses actually play a part in the cancer process, irradiation could prepare the way for them.

Cancer from irradiation can be caused by extremely small doses, though it must be pointed out that it is extremely rare for a single X-ray examination to cause a malignant tumour. However, it has been confirmed that a hundredth of a milligram of radium bromide distributed in the human skeleton causes a malignant tumour. In view of this, subscribers to the mutation theory agree that, in some cases, even a single "direct hit" by radiation can cause a mutation.

Very high doses of radiation do not in any way coincide with a high incidence of cancer. Laboratory studies on young mice, in which some were treated externally with radiation and some internally with radioactive isotopes, produced results that were at first sight bewildering. When the dose of radiation was increased to 350 Röntgen units (r) there was a parallel increase in the frequency of leukaemia. If the dose was increased still further, the frequency of disease fell rapidly.

This seems at first to be paradoxical. It can, nevertheless, be accounted for if it is compared with other statistics, such as the number of surviving cells in an irradiated cell population. This number becomes progressively smaller, the higher the dose given. With increasing dosage, more and more cells are killed or at least so damaged that they lose their ability to multiply. In a comparison of experiments in mice, the late Hal Gray, in Houston,

Texas, succeeded in establishing that the appearance of leukaemia after irradiation depends not only on the increasing number of "direct hits", but also on the similarly increasing number of cells that are killed. Thus, with higher doses, the frequency of leukaemia at first increases in proportion to the increasing number of "direct hits", but falls again as more cells are inactivated or killed.

The frequency of leukaemia therefore depends on the number of hits. At least in young mice a few weeks old, like those used in these experiments, a single "hit" on a cell is not enough to cause malignancy. Only a series of hits leads to the formation of a cancerous tumour.

One or more hits?

Further experiments on mice show, however, that the radiation dose at which the frequency of cancer reaches its maximum falls with increasing age of the animals. Thus, whilst in young mice the climax is reached with a dose of about 350 Röntgens, at which the curve of the frequency of cancer again becomes lower, this dose is reduced in older animals to about 150 Röntgens.

From this it can be concluded that perhaps even a single hit is enough to change the cells of older animals into cancer cells. In this connection, some investigators have formulated an interesting theory. They claim that several "hits" are always necessary to make cells malignant. But cells in older animals, so it is maintained, have already been exposed to other carcinogenic influences in the course of their existence, and therefore a single "hit" by radiation might be enough to make them malignant.

A single high dose of radiation may also cause leukaemia in man. The victims of the atom bomb explosions in Hiroshima and Nagasaki experienced this in the most tragic way. On the other hand, minimal but frequent doses of radiation may have the same effect, as the fate of many radiologists and radiotherapists shows. Although nowadays all conceivable protective measures are taken, sarcoma and leukaemia are much commoner in these professions than in the rest of the population.

Acute leukaemia in children can be traced to irradiation, if their mothers have been exposed to it during pregnancy. An investigation in the United States lasting for more than four years, in which more than a thousand parents and children were involved, gave clear indication that X-ray examinations before pregnancy could later cause leukaemia in the children.

Many of the mothers of 319 children who had leukaemia had undergone X-ray examinations either before or during pregnancy. There were also indications that in some cases X-ray treatment of the father could have played a part.

The research team was able to state that of women examined or treated before pregnancy by X-rays, 60 per cent gave birth to children more prone to leukaemia than those of the other mothers. According to this research, the greatest risk from X-rays is during the last third of pregnancy. The children of women who had previously had a miscarriage, the tests showed, also had a greater tendency to leukaemia.

Children irradiated soon after birth similarly showed a certain vulnerability to leukaemia. If only a part of the body was irradiated, it was comparatively harmless. But children irradiated in several places contracted leukaemia twice as often. The difference between children frequently irradiated and those who had not been irradiated at all was still greater. Those who had been irradiated for an enlarged thymus gland contracted leukaemia three times as often as those in the normal control group. But the fact must also be recognised that the thymus itself may play an important part in leukaemia.

For and against X-rays

Do these startling results imply the end of the X-ray screen in diagnosis? The American medical team who organised that investigation answered this question with a clear NO! "Our results in no way suggest that irradiation should be excluded from medicine. Leukaemia is a comparatively rare disease. The value of irradiation in diagnosis or treatment is much greater than its disadvantages."

In fact, the risk that tuberculosis of the lung may be diagnosed too late, because regular X-ray examinations were foregone, is much greater than the risk of leukaemia or another form of cancer which might be attributable to the X-rays. On the other hand, there is no doubt that irradiation has been carelessly used in the past and that X-ray examinations have frequently been arranged when normal diagnostic methods would have sufficed. The late French research worker, Charles Oberling, did not mince his words. He said: "In all the pessimism about the future of mankind prompted by the advances of our age, one must not forget that the most deadly sources of carcinogenic radiation are not to be found in nuclear plants or bombs, but in the X-ray equipment of our doctors and sanatoria. Immense damage is done here."

In every medical examination by X-rays, Oberling warned, the patient receives a dose of 25 to 30 r. One must remember that there is probably no minimum level of harmfulness, but that 350 r are definitely in the danger zone. Whoever is treated over a period of time for disease of the lungs or similar conditions, usually receives a critical total dose.

Sunlight is also dangerous

Man is not only threatened by X-rays or radioactive substances. About 10 per cent of cancerous diseases can be traced to sources to which man owes his life on this planet; to sunlight or, more precisely, to its ultraviolet spectrum. This is mostly cancer of the skin, because ultraviolet rays do not go very deep. This kind of cancer was first noted in farmers and seamen, and among people employed for many years in the open air. Since brown-tanned faces and bodies have become a general ideal of beauty, "sun cancer" has lost its exclusiveness to certain occupations. The skins of professional sun-worshippers have therefore been thoroughly investigated. This has shown that the parts of the skin exposed to ultraviolet rays become prematurely aged. In addition their liability to cancer increases.

Professor Ward, President of the Australian Dermatological Society, reports that skin cancer in that comparatively sparsely populated continent claims at least one human life every day.

Ninety-five per cent of all cases, Ward thinks, are due to the effect of sunlight that is too strong. Malignant tumours are twenty times more common in Australia than in cloudy England.

In 1925 it was already possible to cause cancer in mice by means of ultraviolet rays. Ordinary sunlight can also cause skin tumours in white rats, for example, if these animals are exposed to the sun over long periods for several hours a day.

People with very pale skin are especially liable to injury by ultraviolet rays. Dark-hued people with skins very rich in pigment are, on the other hand, better protected. Cancer of the skin is rarest in negroes. An exception to this are people suffering from *Xeroderma pigmentosum*, in which there is an abnormal sensitivity of the skin to ultraviolet rays. Usually several parts of the skin are affected by cancer, often in quite young people.

In this instance one can correctly speak of an inheritable disease. Not of inherited cancer, but of an increased liability determined by heredity which leads, almost certainly, to malignant tumours. This poses the question which concerns many people: is cancer inheritable? Is it imposed on certain people from the beginning? The Heidelberg cancer investigator Karl Heinrich Bauer considers this to be "a key question". "Cancer houses" and "cancer families" in which this disease was said to be inherited by one generation from another have, in the past, greatly increased man's fear of cancer. Many early scientists were unable to discount the possibility that cancer is transmitted from generation to generation.

However, this fatalistic view has now been emphatically refuted. Hardly any expert today speaks of direct inheritance of cancer. In the first place, research on identical twins has proved it unlikely. Clearly if the destiny of cancer is predetermined by a hereditary unit in the chromosomes or genes, then people who come from the same fertilised egg, and who are genetically the same, must succumb to the same degree.

But reports by European and American research workers show that this is not at all the case. In Germany it was Otmar von Verschuer who took up the study of twins and cancer with incomparable patience. His last comprehensive research, in 1959, showed that only 34 of 196 identical twins developed cancer more or less simultaneously – a comparatively small number.

Professor K. H. Bauer summed it up. He wrote: "Nothing refutes the thesis of cancer inheritance so much as the spontaneous experiment of twins." If cancer were determined by heredity, twins must, under the direction of their identical chromosome, become ill at the same time, naturally supposing that each twin would be old enough still to experience the cancer "imposed" on it by its genes.

Two doctors, Dr. Lissy F. Jarvik and Dr. Arthur Falek, of the

Psychiatric Institute of New York State, found a still smaller incidence of cancer in twins, of whom they examined more than 1,600. All were over 60 years old and their morbid history was followed for a dozen years. Sixty of them had cancer. And in only three cases had twins that were hereditarily similar both contracted cancer.

If cancer were inherited, then tumours in organs that are identically determined by heredity should be quite common. But the opposite is the case. In the large clinics of the world, cases in which cancer, of, say, both kidneys or both lungs or both sexual glands has been found, are regarded as medical rarities. Even in breast cancer, in 99 per cent of all cases only one breast is affected.

Higher susceptibility is probable

The comforting discovery that cancer is not inherited, either directly or remotely, can consequently be confidently accepted by cancer investigators. But two exceptions must be noted. The relatively rare cases of *Xeroderma pigmentosum* have already been mentioned. The other instance is a cancer of the eye, retinoblastoma. This disease occurs in infancy and was for a long time thought to be incurable. Nowadays 90 per cent of cases of this very rare condition are cured. A predisposition to the disease is clearly transmitted as a dominant factor to the descendants.

Hereditary influences which may lead to a susceptibility to certain forms of cancer seem to be present in many people; such a susceptibility which may possibly be determined by heredity, might lie, among women who develop breast cancer, in disturbances of the hormone metabolism, in an overproduction of the follicle hormone and in a special sensitivity of the mammary gland epithelium. The American cancer investigator Michael B. Shimlin therefore recommended that daughters and sisters of women with breast cancer, and the children of patients with intestinal cancer, should be examined frequently. Professor von Verschuer, too, believed that certain hereditary influences cannot be disregarded in lung cancer.

But, for the rest, what Charles Oberling wrote should be valid: "It is mainly the co-operation of many kinds of anatomical, physiological and immunological conditions determined by heredity, which determines the basis on which cancer can flourish. From this it can be concluded that, with rare exceptions, it is not cancer itself that is inherited, but a combination of conditions which influences and perhaps favours the occurrence of cancer. The transmission of cancer is not the hereditary transmission of a disease, but of a certain constitution."

Among the factors causing cancer, it is highly probable that hereditary tendencies play only a secondary part. They are not the primary cause of cancer, but they favour its origin and promote or inhibit its course. They are not the chief culprits, but accomplices.

The virus theory: the only logical alternative

Charles Oberling – like so many investigators of cancer – died of the disease. He was one of those who most emphatically warned us against regarding cancer as a single disease with a single cause. Whoever thinks that it is enough to discover this cause is making a disastrous error, he said. Even if it should be proved, in the last analysis, that the mechanism of malignant degeneration is the same in all cases, the conditions which lead to it are still very different. After Oberling had been working on cancer for nearly half a century, he concluded that the classical theories of cancer had failed in their endeavour satisfactorily to explain the tumour processes. For him, the virus theory seemed to be "the only logical alternative in the endeavour to reduce all known etiological factors in the causation of cancer to a common denominator".

Chapter 4

VIROLOGISTS – "HOT ON THE TRAIL"

So far the culprit has not been convicted. However, the weight of circumstantial evidence constantly becomes greater. Perhaps it will soon be possible to state that viruses can not only cause cancer in animals, but also in man. As the American cancer investigator Dr. Michael Shimkin said: "The question is no longer whether human cancer is caused by a virus, but which kinds of cancer are to be ascribed to which viruses."

The author heard similar statements in a no less definite form from many other cancer experts. They reflect the complete change that has occurred in the study of cancer during the last 10 to 15 years, at any rate in America. Virology has moved from the perimeter to the centre of cancer investigation. The speed with which science has begun to envelop and unravel the phenomenon of the malignant cell has been determined decisively by the virologists.

For centuries it was otherwise, and belief in the part played by chemical substances and irradiation was long dominant. The existence and effects of human cancer viruses seemed to many incredible or even absurd. In fact, the list of viruses which caused cancer in mice, rats, hens, frogs, apes, hamsters or rabbits continued to grow longer, though most students of virology would not credit such a fact in man. They carefully avoided using the word virus in connection with the causes of cancer. As the American virologist Dr. Bernice Eddy said, "one speaks instead of 'factors', 'influences' or 'unknown substances'."

One of the reasons for this certainly lay in the lamentable bankruptcy of the theory that cancer was, like most other infectious diseases, caused by minute forms of life. This theory was advanced for the first time by the Frenchman Bernard Peyrilhe, in 1775, the year in which Percival Pott had described "chimney sweep cancer". Peyrilhe, a surgeon like Pott, had injected under the skin of a dog some drops of fluid from the breast of a woman with cancer. At the site of the injection there developed a severe inflammation and other symptoms of disease. However, before further observations could be made the dog was drowned by Peyrilhe's assistant, who could no longer bear the animal's illness.

Peyrilhe was not deterred by this from stating, in an essay which later received a prize from the Lyons Academy of Sciences, that human cancer was caused by an infectious agent. The view that cancer may be a transmissible disease carried weight until far into the next century. Many even thought that it must have its origin in a venereal disease. Some hospitals refused to admit patients with cancer; others banished them to separate wings which were strictly isolated.

Ignorance, prejudice and moral presumption branded cancer patients, like syphilitics, with a stigma, the disease being seen as a divine punishment for a dissolute life. In New York a separate cancer hospital had to be built for the treatment and study of this "repulsive disease" which was generally considered to be incurable.

The search for a cancer microbe

In the middle of the 19th century the great era of microbiology, started by Louis Pasteur, began. This was the hour of bacteriology and the microbe hunters. One microbe after another was caught under the objectives of their ever-improving microscopes. One cause of disease after another was identified and overcome with newly-developed chemical preparations. The old scourges of mankind, such as plague, dysentery and cholera, became no more than memories of a dark and ill-civilised chapter in human history. Emil von Behring's diphtheria serum and Robert Koch's tuberculin were the first of the 'magic bullets' by which all diseases were to be eradicated and banished from the earth.

This faith in progress triumphed and scientists seemed more and more to be the wonder men of the age. They cherished great hopes of soon finding a specific cause of cancer. Once the cancer microbe was in the net, the corresponding treatment would soon follow. Over-eager scientists kept announcing victory: unknown bacteria in cancerous tissue were found to be causes of the disease which, it was hoped, would soon be overcome! Always it turned out that these were only additional infections, not cancer microbes. The theory of the bacterial origin of cancer always foundered on the fact that cancer is not infectious. No doctor or nurse had become infected by the tumour of a cancer patient.

Thus it was proved that cancer was not caused by bacteria. Slowly the microbe hunters had to accept this unalterable fact. When once more the tentative conjecture cropped up that not bacteria, but even smaller forms of life must be concerned in the origin of cancer, most experts would not even enter into a discussion of a hypothesis which would probably end up as a similar failure.

One of the last pupils of Pasteur, Amédée Borrel, had, in 1903, expressed this suspicion for the first time in view of the cell growth caused by the smallpox virus. But he remained alone. Many scientists of the orthodox school firmly rejected the existence of such supposedly infinitesimal particles. Unlike bacteria, they could not at that time be made visible under the light microscope. But it could be proved that they were nevertheless present by the roundabout method of filtrates and the infections these caused.

And there was something else. The viruses could not multiply as bacteria do in a test tube on suitable media. They were apparently quite insensitive to cold and to all the available methods of drying. Therefore the question arose whether they were living organisms, or should not rather be regarded as "biological curiosities", a somewhat dubious subject for research by erudite cranks.

Such a crank was the Dutch botanist Willem Beijerinck, Professor at Delft, who had, as a fanatical bachelor, forbidden his assistants to marry – for "a scientist does not marry!" But Beijerinck was, for all that, a brilliant investigator. In 1898 he discovered the activity of the first of these mysterious particles in the tobacco mosaic virus. As a matter of fact, he considered the virus to be not a solid particle, but a fluid which he named "virus", after the mediaeval word "virus" meaning poison.

Action at the Rockefeller Institute

Four years after Borrel had published his thesis, the two Danish investigators Wilhelm Ellermann and Olaf Bang reported that a certain form of leukaemia in hens was caused by a virus.

However, leukaemia and lymphoma were at that time not so strictly categorised as cancer. Three years later the next scene of action was the American Rockefeller Institute. There the pathologist Peyton Rous (now the senior virologist, and 1966 Nobel Prize Laureate for Medicine) had detected a virus which caused sarcoma in hens. Rous, who knew of the work of Ellermann and Bang, investigated the apparently spontaneous tumour in a hen. He found a malignant tumour of the connective tissue, undoubtedly a sarcoma. Rous washed off some pieces of this sarcoma and passed them through a filter which held back the cells and bacteria. Then he injected the cell-free solution into a series of chickens. Some of the animals developed the same characteristic, slowly-growing tumours. They were undoubtedly malignant, as metastases subsequently proved.

Although virology still ranked at that time as a kind of illegitimate offspring of bacteriology, Rous achieved world wide fame through this work – but it did not act as a general stimulus to research. The highest scientific authorities decided that cancer in hens and cancer in man were two quite different matters.

Moreover, experiments with viruses were still undertakings that were as difficult as they were time-consuming. The chief tools of virologists in those days were porcelain filters with tiny pores. It was still impossible to make a single virus visible or to determine its structure and appearance. Hopes that this would change seemed, moreover, decidedly slim. The light microscope had helped bacteriologists to identify one cause of disease after another and ultimately to conquer them with chemotherapeutic weapons. But now it had reached the utmost limit of its efficiency.

The theories of Borrel and Rous, the two "voices crying in the wilderness", first received support in 1933. Dr. Richard Shope who, like Rous, was on the staff of the Rockefeller Institute, found a virus in growths on the skin of a certain species of wild rabbit. This papilloma, named after him, could be transmitted free of cells, either by injection or by application to skin wounds. Some of the wart like growths that were at first benign could later become malignant – in contrast to human warts which are likewise caused by viruses.

Dr. Bittner shocks the experts

Still more important was a discovery made three years later by a young investigator in the Jackson Memorial Laboratory at Bar

Harbour. Dr. John Bittner had found that breast cancer in mice was often caused by a virus which young mice absorbed from their mothers' milk. Bittner, aware of the sad experiences of his predecessors, was exceedingly careful. Carefully he avoided in his thesis the word "virus", to which so many of his colleagues were obviously allergic. Instead he spoke – in face of some ridicule – of a "Milk Factor" in relation to breast cancer of mice.

That was as far as the virologists had got! If they wished to be taken seriously by the rest of the expert world, they had to mask their discoveries in general terms. Bittner himself was convinced that viruses were not the only cause of this mouse-cancer. In his opinion two additional factors – hereditary predisposition and certain hormonal conditions – must be present to cause the disease to become active. The results of later research proved him right.

Bittner had reported on his discovery in extremely cautious terms. But his findings were too important, even too shocking, to permit further research on cancer virus to remain a matter for a few outsiders. In laboratories all over the world the search for cancer viruses was energetically taken up, and special research teams were organised. But new successes proved elusive.

Portrait of a microdwarf

That was clearly not true of many other diseases caused in man and animals by viruses. In the 1930's finer filters and membranes became available to virologists, as well as the first ultracentrifuges and ultimately the electron microscope, which made possible magnification of almost 12,000 times. Now, more and more pathogenic viruses were identified in rapid succession. At last it had become possible to make them visible and to determine their size. Whilst the unit of measurement for bacteriologists was the micron, 1 thousandth of a millimetre, virologists had to add a much smaller unit for the objects they studied, because viruses, in contrast to conventional bacteria, were nothing short of "micro-dwarfs".

The "yardstick" of the virologists became the millimicron, a millionth part of a millimetre. The pox viruses showed themselves to be the largest of all, but they ranked at 200–350 millimicrons, in front of the herpes virus, which measures only 100–175 millimicrons. Still smaller are the myxoviruses (70–120 millimicrons) which cause, for example, influenza and mumps.

Enteroviruses, which cause infantile paralysis as well as diseases of the air passages, are some of the smallest at a size of 20–30 millimicrons.

In 1935 the tobacco-mosaic virus, with which the Dutchman Beijerinck had for the first time proved the existence of viruses, caused more excitement. Dr. Wendell Stanley, an American biochemist, reported a startling experiment which revived the debate as to whether viruses should be regarded as dead or alive.

Stanley was originally – like most biochemists in the thirties – interested in proteins. Three of these proteins, urease, trypsin and pepsin, which acted at the same time as important enzymes in the circulatory system of the human body, had at that time been crystallized. Crystals are formed of single molecules identical with one another, which are attached to each other by their surfaces. If a chemical compound is successfully crystallized, this provides a kind of certificate of purity.

Viruses crystallized

What does the infectious material of a virus consist of? Stanley – and most virologists with him – firmly believed that it must be a protein. The tobacco mosaic virus seemed to be especially suitable for the crystallization of such a virus protein. It provided the best prerequisites. It is stable under all possible conditions, it is easily handled, infected plants can be identified without trouble and it can be obtained in large quantities. Stanley succeeded in crystallising the virus from the sap of barrels of tobacco leaves. It was possible to keep the crystals for as long as he liked, but they could be again dissolved into a fluid without difficulty and without any change in the properties of the virus. But what was much more important: the crystals themselves were a thousand times more infectious than the sap of the tobacco leaves.

For a long time scientists were unable to assess the significance of Stanley's discovery. Apparently lifeless crystals, which should multiply themselves like microbes in another living being – this turned upside down many biologist's general view of life. After a long scientific dispute they drew comfort from a hypothesis which was as plain as it was convenient, that ultimately plant and human viruses may be quite different; as different as the diseases that they respectively cause.

This attitude was not so astonishing. Who suspected at that time that, only a decade after Stanley's experiment, it would be possible to crystallize not only plant viruses but also those that cause the most dangerous human diseases? Thus in 1958 the poliovirus was crystallized, a virus that each year claims many human victims.

Nucleic acids: the heart of the virus

When Stanley succeeded in crystallizing the tobacco mosaic virus, he had, however, overlooked one important fact. The virus crystals did not consist entirely of protein, as he thought. Another still more important substance was concealed in them. The pointer to this was found by the British biochemists Frederick Bawden and Norman Pirie, who repeated Stanley's experiments and discovered phosphorus in the crystals.

Phosphorus does not occur in proteins, but is a constituent of those compounds which mysteriously ensure heredity in every new generation: the nucleic acids. Concealed under a protein covering, the nucleic acid revealed itself as the actual offensive weapon of the virus. Even when the whole virus penetrates into the cells – as has nowadays been proved in many cases – it is only the nucleic acid which takes over the biochemical command. Viruses can infect cells only through their nucleic acid. This was subsequently proved by the brilliant experiments of the German-American Heinz Frankel-Conrat of the University of California.

It was with the tobacco-mosaic virus that infections with pure nucleic acid were first made sucessfully – infections which led to the reformation of complete virus particles in the host cells. It is frequently possible to infect with pure nucleic acid cells which are resistant to the intact virus. This clearly depends on the fact that the antibodies formed by the body's own resistance are adapted only to the protein constituent of the virus.

Research workers have meanwhile clarified to a great extent how the "assumption of power" by viruses occurs in organisms that they infect. The viruses first try to eliminate the DNA of the host cells, but instead, the DNA and RNA of the invader take over the control of the cell. The formation of virus-nucleic acid begins, followed by the formation of virus-protein. When the virus synthesis is completed, or when the activity of the virus has brought about non-physiological conditions in the cell, "lysis" occurs, the cell membrane bursts and thousands of new viruses appear.

The ideal research materials for the study of virus attacks on the cell were at one time almost exclusively the phages. These are a special kind of virus which attack bacteria only. But the modes of infection of viruses which cause diseases in man have also been extensively studied in recent years. This is especially true of the influenza and poliomyelitis viruses.

Since a group of American investigators under the direction of John Franklin Enders succeeded in cultivating the polio virus in tissue culture, the field of knowledge of virology – which even at the end of the fifties was comparable with the state of bacteriology at the time of Robert Koch – has been considerably extended. In many cases virologists have stolen a march even on bacteriologists in terms of detailed knowledge of their field of research.

The two faces of Interferon

The invading virus does not cause the death of the invaded cell in every instance – as does, for example, the polio virus. This is because the cell is not completely helpless against the attack. It produces – as we know today – a protective substance, Interferon, which often re-establishes the equilibrium between the virus and the cell.

The name Interferon was coined by the English scientists Alex Isaacs and Jean Lindenmann. They had in 1957 transferred inactivated influenza virus to embryonic tissue of the chicken and thereby made an astonishing discovery. An acid-resistant substance was formed which, when it was further transferred to other cultures of chicken tissue, inhibited the multiplication of infective influenza virus.

Further investigations showed that Interferon is not only released by inactivated viruses, but also by contact of the cell with infective viruses. But in that case the formation of Interferon is delayed.

Would it perhaps be possible to use Interferon as a weapon for the chemotherapeutic control of virus diseases? Whilst the treatment of bacterial infections by sulphonamides and antibiotics achieved unexpected results, the viruses have so far shown themselves resistant to every kind of chemical attack. The discovery of Interferon now raised hopes among virologists that for once it would be possible to draw level with their colleagues in bacteriology.

Subsequently it has been found that almost all viruses liberate Interferon in the cell. But the amount of Interferon produced varies greatly from one kind of virus to another. But what is still more important: Interferon is not always of the same type. The substances produced by different species of animals actually differ only slightly in their molecular structure, but sufficiently to render the Interferon of one species inactive in another. Furthermore, some viruses are highly sensitive to this protein, while others show a higher resistance to it.

It has now been established that the production of Interferon can be induced not only by viruses, but also by mycoplasmata, Rickettsias and bacteria.

Research with different strains of measle and polio viruses showed that non-virulent strains stimulated the production of Interferon more strongly than virulent strains did. Isaacs therefore took the view that the more virulent a virus is, the less it stimulates the production of Interferon and the more resistant it is to this substance.

Infections with many virulent strains favour the production of proteolytic enzymes in the cell. These enzymes, in turn, break down the Interferon. The virus can then spread rapidly in the affected cell population and destroy it.

An accomplice for viruses?

Naturally, cancer research also busied itself with this inhibitor of virus-destructive activity. What part did Interferon play? Was it on the side of the body in its defence against the cancer viruses, or must it be regarded as an accomplice of the invaders of the cell?

It is clear that in ordinary virus diseases Interferon is an important defence of the cell against infection. It inhibits the multiplication of the viruses and thus hinders the rapid destruction of the cells. But in cancer things are quite different. In this disease the cells are admittedly not destroyed and broken up by the virus. On the other hand, it is characteristic of cancer cells that they are unchecked and go on dividing briskly. When, therefore, the destructive effect of a carcinogenic virus is diminished by Interferon, the malignant cells could perhaps be enabled, by this very effect, to divide further and to develop into a tumour.

Research carried out by Dr. Anthony Clifford Allison, of the National Institute for Medical Research in London, found that the polyoma virus and the Rous-sarcoma virus stimulate the formation of Interferon in cells, though not very strongly. They are also sensitive to Interferon, but less so than many other viruses.

Further experiments showed that the Interferon formed in some tumour cells has only a relatively weak effect. All this seems to point to the fact that the tumour viruses are inhibited by Interferon and do not destroy the cell. Instead, they develop further in the host cell and can change it into a cancer cell.

Allison emphasized that tumour viruses must be able to grow in the host cell, but may not be very virulent. If, for example, a large number of the infected cells are destroyed, or so damaged that they can no longer divide and multiply, then no tumour cells – or only a few groups of them – could develop. But if a large quantity of virus which has been weakened in power is able to persist in the cell, then groups of tumour cells are formed. Possibly, Allison thinks, the Interferon contributes directly to the fact that weakened tumour viruses cause permanent infections.

Interferon is thus two-faced. Whilst it helps the cell to overcome many virus infections, it can, by weakening the tumour viruses, prepare the way for cancer.

Nevertheless it is true that this sphere of research is still in its infancy. Definite conclusions are not yet possible. But virologists will certainly wrest more and more secrets from Interferon.

A paediatrician finds breaks in chromosomes

The whole field of virus research must benefit from this. There are other viruses which do not kill the cell when they attack it, but rather deform the nucleus and cause fragmentation of the chromosomes. In this category for example, is a virus discovered only in 1954, which resembles a tiny horse chestnut with its case and spines. This causes measles, a disease previously classified as one of the harmless ailments of childhood. But since the Swedish paediatrician Dr. Albert Lund discovered chromosome fragments in the blood cells of children suffering from measles, doctors have become very cautious about this disease.

The cells used for the demonstration of chromosomal breakdown are taken from the blood of a child suffering from measles during the febrile stage of the disease. Some of the cells are then artificially cultivated. At the moment when they prepare to divide, the division is artificially arrested by chemical means, or with such alkaloids as colchicin. Then – as when making a blood film – these cells are smeared on to glass slides; deformations of individual chromosomes in the cell nucleus are then clearly visible either under the phase-contrast microscope or the ordinary light microscope. Nowadays, changes or breaks in the chromosomes can be induced artificially in the laboratory.

Optimism in the U.S.A.

We do not yet know the significance of these breaks in the chromosomes, or what their consequences may be. The fact that the breaks have a fatal similarity to the chromosomal changes found in people suffering from leukaemia, has greatly puzzled scientists. This discovery has revived the hitherto open question as to whether viruses may also play an active part in human cancer.

Many European scientists still react to this question with an uncomfortable shrug of the shoulders. The reaction is different in the United States. Most American investigators of cancer also give a qualified answer, but many of them bluntly concede in private conversation that, in leukaemia at least, certain viruses must be considered as "highly suspect". Many Americans are even convinced that conclusive proof of guilt will soon be found, and that the manufacture of corresponding vaccines may be near at hand. This led the President of the American Cancer Society, Dr. Wendell Scott, at the end of 1964 to the rather rash prophecy that "in two years at the latest, leukaemia will be struck off the list of incurable diseases".

This development caused the American Congress, in 1964, to set aside another 10 million dollars for a special programme of research into the relationship between leukaemia and viruses. The Congress Committee concerned also declared, after hearing the highest scientific authorities, "the virus origin of leukaemia is very near the stage of complete scientific proof".

With the additional 10 million dollars, the amount of money invested in the United States in cancer research in 1965 had grown to almost 400 million dollars!

The fact that viruses have again become the focus of cancer research is due to some sensational discoveries made by a number of scientists in the last 10 years. None of them has yet been able to specify a certain virus or group of viruses as the cause of cancer in man, but the chain of circumstantial evidence is constantly becoming more complete. As Dr. Franz Josef Rauscher, of the National Cancer Institute, explained; "there are too many related facts to permit us to ignore the virus theory in the future. I am firmly convinced that a virus plays at least a part in human leukaemia."

This Cancer Institute is one of the five new research centres combined into the impressive complex of laboratories of the National Institutes of Health near Washington. About 600 scientists and assistants work in the Cancer Institute. When it was founded in 1937 by a resolution of Congress it had at its disposal a budget of 400,000 dollars. Today its annual expenditure amounts to more than 140 million dollars. Only 20 per cent of this sum, however, is used directly for the work of the Institute itself. 80 per cent of the fund allocated by the Government is made available to universities throughout the country for cancer research.

Industrial firms are also given contracts by the Institute if they work on the discovery or testing of new anti-cancer drugs.

In its special leukaemia programme, the National Cancer Institute co-operates closely with the drug firm of Pfizer, which has today undertaken the preparatory work for a leukaemia vaccine. This involves, in the first place, the cultivation of great quantities of virus material needed for the subsequent manufacture of the vaccine. Viruses for this purpose have already been produced in considerable quantities, and have been successfully kept alive.

Rauscher, now 35 years old, is chief of the virus investigation programme of the National Cancer Institute. He has discovered a virus (now named after him) which causes a rapid enlargement of the spleen in certain animals. It either kills them or causes them to contract leukaemia. Rauscher is one of the most consistent advocates of the theory that leukaemia in man is also caused by a virus. "Virus may also play a part in cancer of the breast and genital organs," he says.

But why, if this is so, have no cancer viruses been found as the causes of human tumours? Such a question overlooks the fact that, in human tumours, there is a latent period of up to several decades. If a virus were the cause of cancer, the first contact between this virus and the cell would have to be made in the unborn child in the womb or in early childhood. The virus nucleic acids would then be transmitted continuously as a kind of additional gene in the divisions of the cancer cells.

Viruses cannot always be isolated from animal tumours, even with their much shorter latent periods. The usual method rather provides indirect proof of them. A cell-free extract is obtained from the tumour tissue and is inoculated into other animals. These animals – if the virus theory is correct – develop identical tumours. Such experiments, which involve a risk of death, are naturally forbidden in man.

Perhaps viruses which cause human cancer have already been photographed. Dr. Leon Dmochowski of the Anderson Hospital at the University of Texas probably has the most comprehensive collection of pictures of viruses ever made with the electron microscope. Several of them show virus-like particles found in different kinds of cancer cells – of animals and man. For the most part, these virus particles could not be found in healthy cells. But in some cases Dmochowski found them also – admittedly in small numbers – in the cells of animals which were susceptible to cancer but had not yet developed it. He created the greatest sensation by his discovery of suspicious particles in the milk of mice, and women, suffering from breast cancer.

Research success in an Army Hospital

After the Second World War, Dr. Ludvik Gross, of the Army Administration Hospital in the Bronx district of New York, gave the decisive impulse to cancer virology. Gross, an emigrant from Poland, is the type of investigator who becomes completely absorbed in his work. In heavily-accented English he reports: "My interest in cancer originated in Europe, when I was able – as a young surgeon – to study my first cases of cancer. They were tumours of the lips in pipe-smoking peasants and cancers of the skin – almost always a picture of horrible devastation of the cells."

Gross turned to internal medicine and later, during the Second World War, began to investigate cancer in the Army Hospital. He concentrated upon a strain of mice, of which many "spontaneously" developed leukaemia in the early months of life.

In 1956 Gross gave the death blow to this theory. He proved that the disease never appeared "spontaneously". On the contrary, it was clearly caused by a virus.

Gross showed this in the following way. He obtained an extract from the organs of animals suffering from leukaemia. The cell-free filtrate of this extract was then inoculated into newly-born mice of a strain that showed a very low incidence of "spontaneous" leukaemia. After the inoculation, a high percentage of these mice developed leukaemia. When further animals were inoculated with the filtrate, its carcinogenic effect was increased considerably. Gross was now able to induce leukaemia in all newly-born mice.

"Wanted" notice for a mouse virus

Gradually Gross succeeded in making out a "wanted" notice for this virus. It is a particle with a diameter of about 100 millimicrons, which easily passes through all filters impenetrable by bacteria. The virus is relatively sensitive to heat, and is inevitably destroyed if exposed to about 50 degrees C. for 30 minutes. But in solid carbon dioxide, at a temperature of – 70 degrees, it can easily be stored and maintained intact. It can be bred in tissue cultures, for instance, on normal mouse embryo cells. The fluid from such cultures, kept in test tubes for some weeks at a temperature of 37 degrees, can still cause leukaemia if it is injected into newly-born mice. Normally the leukaemia virus is transmitted from the parents to their offspring.

Other investigators succeeded, after Gross, in isolating viruses that cause leukaemia in mice. The American virologist Charlotte Friend, of the Sloan-Kettering Institute, based her work not on leukaemia, but on cell-free extracts of the Ehrlich tumour. The virus in this caused leukaemia two weeks after injection into adult mice.

The Director of the Institute for cancer research in Berlin-Buch, Professor Arnold Graffi, obtained a similar virus from carcinomas and sarcomas of mice. This virus not only caused leukaemia in mice, but also tumours in the thoracic cavity of newly-born rats.

Presumably leukaemia viruses exist in the cells of many normal mice. They are transmitted from one generation to another. These vertical infections only rarely result in an outbreak of disease. "It is quite possible," says Gross, "that normal and completely healthy animals harbour viruses not only of leukaemia, but also of tumours. The latent viruses behave as parasites, content with their modest demands, without causing in their host any detectable injury. Suddenly they are stimulated into action. They change from harmless parasites into pitiless causes of disease."

The activated viruses can drive their host cells to rapid multiplication. According to the type by which the organism is infected, the development of leukaemia or tumours results.

It had scarcely been established that apparently spontaneous leukaemia in a certain strain of mice was really the work of viruses, when another report alarmed cancer investigators. This time it came from two ladies, the virologists, Dr. Sarah Stewart and Dr. Bernice Eddy.

Sarah Stewart, like Rauscher, was originally a bacteriologist. At first she set about examining Dr. Ludvik Gross's work on leukaemia. To do this, she obtained from Gross mice of the strain he was using. And she came upon an astonishing fact: the mice contained not just one virus, but two different types. One of these did, in fact, cause leukaemia. The other caused the formation of solid tumours, not only in the spleen, as was first thought, but also in almost all the organs of mice, rats, and hamsters.

This virus, like the leukaemia virus, became steadily more malignant after Dr. Stewart had succeeded, with her colleague Dr. Eddy, in cultivating it further in various laboratory cultures. Altogether this type of virus could cause about 20 different forms of cancer. It therefore rightly bore its name of Polyoma virus ("many tumour virus").

Graffi discovered another polyoma virus. He named this after the location of his Institute "T/2 Berlin-Buch". "We were working at that time on mouse leukaemia" he says. "By transmitting the leukaemia virus we induced leukaemia in about 80 per cent of the mice. On the other hand, about 10 per cent of the animals developed solid tumours. As our aim was to cultivate the leukaemia virus, these tumours did not at first interest us at all. They merely disturbed us.

"When Stewart and Eddy isolated a polyoma virus from the

leukaemia mice we naturally became interested. Ultimately we were able to discover a new polyoma-virus, different from the American one. It is the first, and so far the only, virus to cause sarcoma not only in rats, mice, hamsters and guinea pigs, but also in rabbits."

Graffi, however, does not think that there are causal relationships between the leukaemia viruses of mice and polyoma viruses. "It seems more likely that leukaemia cells serve as especially good nutrient media for the polyoma viruses, which are latent in almost all mice."

Further experiments showed that a complete virus is by no means necessary to cause morbid changes in cells and tumours. In 1960 Aaron Bendich, Sarah Stewart and Bernice Eddy succeeded in causing infections in the cells of tissue cultures with pure nucleic acids obtained from mouse cells infected with polyoma virus.

The "naked" nucleic acids also caused tumours in animals – although with less certain results. Some time later the mysterious relationship between nucleic acids and cancer again became evident. DNA isolated from the Shope papilloma virus was able to cause infections without the rest of the virus.

Two further discoveries have recently enabled subscribers to the virus theory to gain new ground. In 1957 American scientists discovered a new group of viruses, which, because they originated from cultures made from the kidney cells of monkeys, were called simian viruses, or S.V. for short.

At first cancer investigators were not greatly interested. These viruses were apparently not malignant, and remained latent in their natural hosts. The SV.40 virus discovered in 1960 was found to be of "good behaviour" in the cells of rhesus and cynomolgus monkeys. But in cell cultures from so-called "green monkeys" (*Cebus callitrichus*), which come from equatorial East Africa, the virus caused remarkable injuries. Moreover, the electron microscope showed that it had a fatal similarity to the versatile polyoma virus.

Hidden in the vaccine

These results sounded a grave warning to virologists: the kidneys of rhesus monkeys were used as the main breeding grounds of poliomyelitis viruses. The viruses thus obtained were used in the fight against infantile paralysis, either as inactivated suspensions for injections or in an attenuated form for oral absorption. If it was true – and of this there could soon be no doubt – that the SV.40 virus was concealed in almost all these kidney cultures, then, in polio inoculations millions of adults and children were simultaneously inoculated with SV.40. It must have been present in the Sabin-polio-vaccines, which contained an attenuated but living virus, and also in the Salk vaccine made from dead polio-viruses. For SV.40 is hardly affected by formaldehyde, with which the polio-virus was attenuated.

Quite soon SV.40 viruses were found in the throats and stools of children inoculated against infantile paralysis. Now the disquieting question arose: what effects could this SV.40 virus produce in man?

Even before a clear answer to this was found, a new discovery shocked virologists: Dr. Bernice Eddy, co-discoverer of the polyoma virus, now investigated the simian viruses. "The idea came to me that some of these viruses could be oncogenic." She herself reports the beginning of her work.

"It was originally my intention to investigate all the known simian viruses to find out if they cause tumours in hamsters. But when I began my work in June, 1959, the list of these viruses had already become too long, and I therefore chose a simpler method.

"I started from the idea that all cell cultures from the kidneys of rhesus monkeys contained one or more simian viruses. Two different cultures of such cells were therefore prepared. After cell growth had become established, the cultures were put into the incubator for 14 days. At the beginning and end of the first week the nutritive fluids were renewed.

"At the end of the second week" continues Dr. Eddy, "90–95 per cent of the fluid was poured off and the cell-residue was separated out by centrifugation. The cells remaining in the experimental flasks were recovered from the glass wall by repeated freezing and thawing. Then this suspension and the cell residue obtained from the fluid were put into a mortar, cooled with dry ice, and ground in the frozen state to a fine powder. The material was then thawed and ultimately injected subcutaneously into the cheek pouches of new-born hamsters."

For four months, no morbid changes were observed in the hamsters. The animals flourished splendidly. But on the 118th day one hamster showed a tumour at the injection site. By the

139th day the same thing had happened in seven other hamsters, and by the 449th day tumours had developed at the injection sites in 20 of the 23 experimental animals. The tumours proved, in subsequent experiments, to be transmissible to other hamsters.

Naturally it was ensured in all tests that the hamsters could not be infected from other sources. Care was also taken to see that no polyoma virus, the oncogenic activity of which was already known, was present in the material from the rhesus kidneys.

Dr. Eddy's experiments had, of course, not yet explained which virus had caused the tumours in the hamsters. In June 1960 the Americans William H. Sweet and Maurice Hilleman discovered that the SV.40 virus caused morbid changes in cell cultures from the African "green monkeys". Dr. Eddy was provided with this virus strain by Dr. Hilleman and she injected it into new-born hamsters. Most of these animals developed tumours which were in distinguishable from those obtained by injection of the extract from the kidneys of rhesus monkeys. Ultimately, Eddy and her colleagues succeeded in isolating from the hamster tumours a new virus, A 426, which proved to be identical with SV.40.

Although a nation-wide campaign for protective inoculation against polio was in progress, the American health authorities and the makers of vaccines responded immediately: manufacture was stopped and comprehensive researches were started into the effects of the SV.40 viruses. Almost all the large virological institutes in the U.S.A. occupied themselves with this urgent task. At the same time work went on to find chemical compounds with which the SV viruses could be killed with certainty.

Common cold in man – cancer in animals

In the course of these feverish investigations the second surprise came – the effect of human viruses on animals.

Dr. John Trentin and his colleagues of the Baylor University in Houston, Texas, had specialised for many years on the adeno-viruses. These were so named because they were first isolated (in 1953) from growths in the adenoids of man. During the next 10 years, more than thirty different adeno-viruses were classified. In man these viruses seem to cause only the harmless symptoms of the common cold. But in 1962 Trentin was able to prove that Type 12 of these viruses were carcinogenic – not in man, but in hamsters. When adeno-virus 12 was injected into young hamsters it caused cancer in most of them.

This observation was verified and expanded in the same year, when Dr. Robert J. Huebner, of the National Institute for Research into allergies and infectious diseases in the U.S.A., found that adeno-viruses of Type 18 also caused cancer in young hamsters. Ultimately two more oncogenic adeno-viruses, Nos. 7 and 31 were added to the list.

But this was not all: in 1965 it was necessary also to add adeno-virus 3. Adeno-virus 4, on the other hand, seems not to be carcinogenic; at any rate, research on hundreds of animals over many years has provided no evidence of this.

Adeno-virus 3 needs a long time before it causes tumours. The type of virus used by Huebner's research team came from the throat of a child who had had a severe cold. After the virus had undergone seven passages through tissue cultures of human cells, Huebner injected it into the skin of new-born hamsters. A long wait began. Only after 275 days did a tumour become noticeable at the injection site in one of the eight animals treated. If the virus material was injected simultaneously under the skin and into the abdominal cavity, tumours developed after 151 days in one of 17 animals.

Huebner estimates that about half of all American children are already infected with adeno-virus 3 before they are 10 years old. Antibodies against this type of virus are present in 70 per cent of all adults. This may be regarded as a certain sign of an earlier or still existing infection.

In view of this "omnipresence", this virus merits the greatest attention, although it apparently causes no more than a common cold in man.

The SV.40 virus under further observation

The SV.40 virus, which contaminated the early polio-vaccines, could not, however, be detected in a single case of human cancer. Although virologists were much relieved, this clearly could not constitute a general "acquittal" of the charge of cancer. Many years of intensive observations will be necessary to be absolutely sure. For in tissue cultures of human cells the SV.40 virus can cause injuries which bear the fatal imprint of malignity: a discovery which has interested many scientists who have hitherto been sceptical about a virus etiology in human cancer.

The American Nobel Prize Laureate John F. Enders, who helped to develop some of the most important vaccines, was able for the first time to breed the SV.40 virus in tissue culture. In order to prepare the cultures, Enders and his colleagues used human embryos from miscarriages, or tissues taken from stillborn children. In this way it was shown that the virus can grow in almost any kind of tissue, and can cause severe injury to the cells in them. Moreover, it was possible to note a pronounced stimulation of growth in many cells.

Although virologists for the time being remain unable to provide definite proof, much importance must be attached to the fact that a virus has been found which is pathogenic to man and causes cancer in animals.

Human cancer transmitted to monkeys

Those opponents of the virus theory who, in view of such discoveries, sought comfort in the fact that there is an infinite difference between man and hamsters, were soon disturbed to find this contention considerably shaken. In 1963 Dr. Michael Epstein of the Middlesex Hospital, London, succeeded in transmitting a human tumour to monkeys. This was a tumour which appeared chiefly in the jaws of children and juveniles, and had first been described by the English expert on tropical diseases, Dennis Burkitt. The particular geographical distribution of this tumour in a climatically defined area of Africa, had suggested that it was caused by a virus transmitted by insects.

Epstein had obtained fresh cells from the glands of a girl affected by the Burkitt lymphoma. He then injected these cells into the abdominal cavity of four young African monkeys. Some years later three of these monkeys were examined and malignant cells were found in their bone marrow, the typical picture of the Burkitt cancer. These cancer cells were then injected into eleven other monkeys, of which five showed, after a relatively short time, the same bone marrow features as their two predecessors.

Apparently human cancer has thus been transmitted to monkeys for the first time, for it is highly improbable that the injected cells had survived and multiplied in the abdominal cavities of the monkeys. As everyone knows, it is difficult enough to keep alive tissue transmitted from one human being to another; it can be taken as certain that human tissues and cells could not exist in the bodies of another species. Therefore an invisible virus, which caused degeneration in the monkey cells, must have been transmitted on that occasion.

The fact that the formation of degenerate cells in the monkeys did not take place until two years after the injections seemed, to the English journal "The New Scientist", to explain why it has not so far been possible to cause cancer in animals by means of human leukaemia cells.

As has already been mentioned, the suspicion has arisen that cancer, especially leukaemia, may be caused by a virus. In the United States 2,500 children die each year of this cancer of the blood-forming tissue. "The trail has become hot" say American scientists, speaking of the earliest discoveries in this field. Since the significant results obtained by Gross, Stewart, Eddy and others, it is an established fact that at least five different kinds of virus can cause leukaemia in mice.

Formerly such research in man was quite impossible. But many things indicate that, in certain circumstances, it may soon be otherwise. Suspicious particles have recently been found in the blood plasma of one of of three children suffering from leukaemia. They had a puzzling similarity to the corresponding mouse viruses. At the same time, human leukaemia cells were successfully cultured in the laboratory for the first time. Dr. James Grace, of the Roswell Park Memorial Institute in Buffalo, found virus-like particles in these cells.

Grace is one of the best-known American immunologists. Since his two-year-old son died of leukaemia he and his wife, who is also a scientist, have devoted themselves with great energy to the investigation of this disease.

Leukaemia cells in the test tube

Grace worked for five years to cultivate leukaemia cells from human patients in test tubes. "First we used the standard method of making cell cultures in glass vessels." he said. "This culminated some weeks later in an excessive growth of fibroblasts, the normal connective tissue cells. Only considerably later and by accident did we discover, during microscopical investigation, that the leukaemia cells do not grow in the bottom of the vessel but in the nutrient medium which had been poured away. It was thus only necessary to change the vessels frequently, and each time to remove the fibroblasts."

In February, 1964, Grace was able to report for the first time on the successful cultivation of leukaemia cells *in vitro*. The first of these cells came from a 78-year-old patient with leukaemia, the next from a 5-year-old child, then from a juvenile and, finally, from a 4-year-old. All these were cases of acute leukaemia. The 78-year-old patient died soon after the experiment.

But her cells had become, in a sense, "immortal". They continue to live on and to multiply in cell cultures in the Roswell Park Memorial Institute and in many other institutes supplied with cultures from Buffalo. Today there are in the world about 20 different cell-lines from various leukaemia patients. In 14 out of 18 of these lines, virus-like particles have been found. "These particles have also been found in about 10–15 per cent of leukaemia patients," reports Grace. "It is extremely difficult to make them visible. Our experimental technique still imposes very narrow limits. Often investigations on the same patient have different results. But such particles have never been found in healthy human beings."

Antigens specific to leukaemia can be found in 50–60 per cent of the patients. It is still not certain whether these consist of virus-like particles or other substances.

The answer in six months . . .

Grace concedes: "We have still much to do before we can prove conclusively that the particles we have found and cultivated are actually viruses, and that they represent the cause of leukaemia. Like all investigators of cancer, we face the problem that our experiments on animals cannot be applied to new-born human beings. If similar restrictions applied to experiments on animals, leukaemia viruses in mice and other animals would hardly have been discovered today. To put it another way: if we could transmit our virus particles to man, we should know inside six months whether or not there are human leukaemia viruses."

At about the same time as Grace in Buffalo, Dr. G. Negroni succeeded in obtaining a new kind of micro-organism from the bone marrow of leukaemic children. Negroni and his colleagues in the London Imperial Cancer Institute indentified this, too, as a virus-like particle. Here again, the classical proof that these particles actually cause leukaemia was naturally not possible. For this, it would have been necessary to infect healthy human beings.

The scientists therefore infected tissue cultures of human cells. The result was that the virus-like particles multiplied in the cultures and damaged the cells. In addition it was shown that the blood serum of leukaemia patients contained special antibodies, which can protect the cultured cells from these virus particles.

Pigmy bacteria form a fifth column

Other investigators reduced the original hopes of the London research team to nothing. They received an investigated Negroni's tissue cultures. They were able to establish that the particles were, without doubt, a species of micro-organism.

In contrast to viruses, this micro-organism could be cultivated on ordinary agar. Dr. R. J. Fallon, Pathologist to the Ruchill Hospital in Glasgow, together with workers from other laboratories therefore postulated that the new cause belonged to the group of Mycoplasms. These are a kind of pygmy bacteria – tiny forms of life which come between bacteria and viruses (PPLO = Pleuropneumonia-like organisms).

These mycoplasms have a much more complicated structure than viruses – they have a stronger protein envelope, and their own metabolism with a corresponding enzyme system. The mycoplasms from Negroni's tissue cultures are about four times as big as the supposed leukaemia viruses.

At present there are two explanations to choose from. One is that the mycoplasms are only additional micro-organisms that somehow got into Negroni's cultures and that virus-like particles are additionally present. The other possibility is that the mycoplasms are the true causes of leukaemia. But they appear in different forms. Perhaps the particles observed by Negroni and his colleagues are fragments of mycoplasms which look like viruses. If this is so, further research work will be much easier, since mycoplasms can be cultivated in cell-free cultures.

Records of mycoplasms in tumour tissues must, however, be examined with care. Dr. Dietmar Gericke, director of cancer research in the Farbwerke Hoechst, emphasizes that they should not lead us to hasty conclusions. Especially where tissue cultures *in vitro* are concerned, the results must be interpreted very critically. The risk of a subsequent infection of the tissue cultures by mycoplasms is so great that the quota of error can amount to 80 per cent.

Dr. Gericke reports, "We have examined 79 human tumours removed by operation and have not found mycoplasms in a single one. In leukaemia patients we have, on the other hand, found these micro-organisms in the blood and also in the bone marrow. However, it must not be forgotten that the resistance of patients with leukaemia is distinctly lowered." They are therefore very susceptible to infections of all kinds, whilst healthy people can only be infected with mycoplasms if extremely high doses of them are given.

Gericke holds it to be very improbable that cancer can be caused by mycoplasms alone. He thinks that a far more interesting question is whether these organisms are co-carcinogenic. If such a hypothesis should be proved, possibilities of prevention might result.

At present, by experiments on animals, the Hoechst laboratories are testing to see whether a mycoplasm infection occurs in the uterus, at a time when the immune tolerance of the body is still very high. If this is so, such infections could be prevented under certain conditions, perhaps by treatment of the mother during pregnancy with tetracyclines, antibiotics which successfully attack mycoplasms.

"Whatever part mycoplasms might play in the cancer process," thinks Dr. Grace of the Roswell Park Memorial Institute, "we can no longer ignore them. They demand new efforts of research."

Cancer viruses are "ordinary" viruses

Virus research in particular goes on in the U.S.A. at high pressure. One fact is already certain: cancer viruses are not basically different from other viruses. Dr. Maurice Hilleman states, "Their most striking feature is their normality". Most of these viruses are structurally quite similar to other viruses. They either contain DNA as does the polyoma virus, or RNA as does the Rous-sarcoma virus. The formation of RNA is, it is thought, controlled by DNA. It is discharged into the cytoplasm in order to control the formation of proteins there.

There are, however, indications of certain differences between the structure of the DNA in ordinary viruses and in those that cause cancer. Dr. Maurice Green, Director of the Institute for Molecular Biology in the University of Philadelphia, has provided important evidence of this. Viruses which cause cancer in experimental animals contain 49 per cent of guanine and cytosine (two of the four bases in DNA), whilst these sub-units amount to 56 per cent in viruses that do not cause cancer.

The significance of this statement is at present still not clear. It may possibly be explained by the fact that the guanine-cytosine portion in cancer viruses more closely resembles the corresponding portion in the DNA of animal cells than does that in other viruses.

Viruses with different kinds of nucleic acids – does this mean that, in the causation of cancer, DNA and RNA attack by different routes? DNA-viruses evidently cause cancer by combination with the DNA of the host. The false information thus imposed on the host DNA is automatically taken up by the RNA, which is formed by a kind of reprint from the DNA-matrix. This leads to alterations in the heredity-structure of the cell, and explains why the descendants of the first malignant cells are also given this genetic defect.

Inheritance by biological feed-back

But it is otherwise with viruses which contain RNA. Naturally an RNA-virus can falsify the RNA code – even more directly than can a DNA particle. This falsification can occur in the cytoplasm, where the RNA controls the protein synthesis. In this way the change of the affected cell into a cancer cell could occur. Because, however, the hereditary structure of the DNA is not affected by this, the RNA formed from the DNA would again contain correct information. The transmission of malignant properties to increasing generations of daughter cells would therefore be conceivable only if it were possible for the altered RNA to affect the DNA by biological feedback.

Thanks to the most recent researches of two Americans, Renato Dulbecco of the Californian Institute of Technology and Harry Rubin of the University of California, the way in which cancer is caused by viruses has become much clearer. Dulbecco found that viruses can make cells malignant without themselves having to multiply. When the DNA of the virus combines with the DNA of the cell, the genetic apparatus is altered, the normal course of cell division is disturbed, and uncontrolled cell growth is caused; this becomes increasingly malignant with each of the subsequent cell generations. The multiplication of the chromosomes no longer proceeds in a disciplined manner, and a kind of natural selection sees to it that a majority of malignant cells remain, with increasingly serious results for the organism.

In this manner, the effect of the virus is transmitted, long after the original infection, to subsequent generations of cells. The incorporated virus-gene is perfectly adequate for this.

It is quite otherwise with RNA viruses. In the Rous-sarcoma of hens, for example, caused by the Rous-sarcoma virus (consisting of RNA), there are infectious and non-infectious tumours. This fact was thoroughly investigated by Harry Rubin. He made the surprising discovery that the virus had, so to speak, a "defect", It was indeed able to cause cell malignancy, but could not give rise to infectious progeny.

To do this it needed an "assistant virus", which is found alongside the Rous-sarcoma virus. This "auxiliary force" first provides the sarcoma virus with the necessary protein envelope; only then is the complete virus able to infect cells and to multiply itself. Both malignant changes in cells and also multiplication of the virus can now occur.

A dangerous defect

Rubin even assumed that there is, in tumour viruses, a deeper relationship between such a "defect" and the ability of the virus to change a normal cell into a malignant one. All viruses known to be able to transmit genetic characteristics from one bacterium to another have, so Rubin says, this defect. In them part of the equipment of heredity is replaced by a segment of the bacterial chromosome. The functions of the genes thus substituted must now be taken over by an assistant virus. Only in this way can the original virus reproduce itself and retain its infectious properties.

It is therefore necessary to find out whether, in the Rous-sarcoma virus, a part of the mechanism of inheritance is replaced by heredity structures of the host cell. Since this virus, however, consists not of DNA, but of RNA, it is more probable that the "defect" arises by a mutation.

The most recent results of research make it increasingly clear why no cancer viruses have yet been found in human tumours. Or rather why, in the case of viruses encountered in tumours, it has not been possible to determine whether they are the causes of the tumours or only harmless parasites. It is probable that cells which are already malignant no longer contain any complete viruses. Their nucleic acid has, wedded itself, in a true "mésalliance", to the nucleic acid of the cells and has become a constituent of the genetic apparatus.

"The true cell parasite," said the late French investigator, Professor Charles Oberling, "is not the whole virus but its nucleic acid, which cannot be separated from the nucleic acid of the cell, and therefore cannot be identified." But the genetic code falsified by the nucleic acid of the virus is transmitted to generations of daughter cells.

Search for an extra DNA molecule

Yet how can it be determined whether the cancer cell contains a nucleic acid molecule added by a virus, or perhaps only some additional nucleotide sequences? Scientists are still not even agreed about the possible number of nucleic acid molecules per individual cell. Estimates vary from 500,000 to more than a million. "How shall we therefore detect an extra molecule?" asks Dr. Bendich of the Sloan-Kettering Institute. "And even if we found such a molecule, we should still be a long way from our goal. How could it be proved that it was actually *this* DNA molecule that effected the change into a cancer cell?"

Bendich and his colleagues have not allowed themselves to be discouraged by such difficulties. They are at present investigating how the nucleic acid of a virus penetrates into the chromosomes and thus into the genetic apparatus. Bendich and his assistant Dr. Ellen Borenfreund have already traced this nucleic acid into the cell nucleus.

The viral origin of cancer is conceivable not only as the interpolation of an additional nucleic acid molecule into the DNA, but also, so many scientists consider, by the reverse process, in which viruses lead to the loss of certain parts of the cell-DNA. The fact that many cancer cells lose part of their antigens under the influence of viruses is additional evidence for this admittedly vague hypothesis.

Many viruses exist in a latent state, and may only be provoked into oncogenic action by special factors. Dr. Francisco Duran-Reynolds, the Spanish-Amerinçan scientist and "cancer-virologist" at a time when cancer viruses were discussed by many scientists as biological chimaeras, was one of the first to demonstrate the part played by chemical influences in this respect. He proved that a certain virus caused cancer if the subjects were treated beforehand with certain chemicals. Neither the virus nor the chemicals were able to do this alone.

Dr. Paul Kotin, formerly of the University of South California and now in the National Cancer Institute, was able to cause lung cancer in mice if he exposed these animals simultaneously to influenza virus and to the fumes of benzole derivatives. Here, too, neither the virus nor the benzole derivatives were able to do this alone. Did the chemical compounds initially provide the requirements which enabled the virus to begin its malignant work?

A series of experiments suggest that irradiation may stir cancer viruses out of their latency. Mice were irradiated to the point when leukaemia was caused; astonishingly this leukaemia was transmissible. With cell-free extracts – this is especially noteworthy – of their tissues it was possible to cause the same disease again in other mice. Only one conclusion is possible from this: the cancer viruses already present in the mice were actuated by the preceding irradiation, and were later transmitted to the other animals in the cell-free extracts. The American investigator Henry Kaplan, and his colleagues, were able to cause cancer by irradiation in a certain strain of mice *only* when the cells of these animals already harboured leukaemia viruses. But clearly the irradiation was necessary to make these viruses carcinogenic.

"Time bombs" in the shape of latent viruses

Yet another example exists in this category. It is known that the number of leukaemia victims rose steeply among the survivors of the atom bomb explosions in Hiroshima and Nagasaki. But if one examines the figures more closely, one finds, as things are at present, that of all the people exposed to the highest doses of radiation, only one in a hundred has acquired leukaemia. Why not the others? Many investigators believe that the effect of radiation was not in itself enough. Perhaps an additional factor is needed to cause the disease. Is this additional factor a virus? If

Dr. Kenneth M. Endicott, Director of the National Cancer Institute in the U.S.A., has his way, we shall soon know. In April 1966, Endicott told a Committee of the American Congress that it may only be a question of time before proof exists that viruses cause some forms of cancer. Endicott considers that the successful attempt to cultivate, in test-tubes, human cancer cells which produce virus particles, would be an important step along the way.

But even if the first cancer viruses are one day discovered in the cells of people who are ill, not every infection need automatically lead to cancer. Dr. James Grace, in a conversation with the author at the Roswell Park Memorial Institue, said: "The disease which follows an infection may very well be the exception, as in infantile paralysis or meningitis. Here the disease occurs after infection with the corresponding virus only once in about 10,000 cases." Many viruses which start the malignant process with almost mathematical precision in laboratory investigations, remain completely inactive in animals living in their natural environment. These "pacifist" cell parasites only change into malignant aggressors after repeated passages through tissue cultures and after transmission to other kinds of animals.

Dr. Ludvik Gross, the discoverer of the leukaemia viruses in mice, is also of this opinion. "Presumably only a small percentage of people who are infected under certain conditions with carcinogenic viruses, become ill," he says. "The others live, as it were, with a time-bomb in their pockets."

Chapter 5

FROM RED-HOT IRONS TO THE LASER BEAM

For more than two thousand years the battle against cancer has been the province of the surgeons. Hippocrates, in the 5th century B.C., burnt out a cancer of the throat with a red hot iron; in 1882 Theodor Billroth removed for the first time the stomach of a woman afflicted with cancer; Harvey Cushing was the first to attempt brain operations; Evarts Graham performed the first successful operations for cancer of the lung and himself died of this disease. They and many other surgeons made the landmarks in the operative treatment of the tumours.

The introduction of blood transfusion, prophylaxis against infections by means of antibodies, heart and lung machines, artificial kidneys and artificial bones and blood vessels, as precursors of transplantations of whole organs, have all helped to improve the armoury against cancer.

Cancer operations rank among the highest levels of surgery. They demand perfect technique and skilful judgment. Such operations are chiefly entrusted to the most experienced specialists.

In contrast to emergency operations, those on cancer are mainly performed on older people whose general condition is often greatly weakened by the disease. These factors necessitate careful preparation and thorough post-operative treatment.

In addition, cancer operations are usually much more extensive and radical than surgical operations of other kinds. When possible, not only must the tumour itself be removed, but also the surrounding tissue in which cancer cells may have begun their fatal dissemination. Every malignant cell remaining in the neighbourhood of the visible tumour must be included. Failing this, new centres of cancer may be formed long afterwards, making further operations necessary. As Karl Heinrich Bauer emphasizes "In the hands of the specialist the more radical operation is always the better one." It alone offers the chance of a permanent cure.

The decision as to whether a tumour is operable or not lays great responsibility on the surgeon. The state of the disease is a decisive factor here. If a large number of secondary tumours have been formed and widely distributed in the body, the operation may at best bring only a short-term respite from the disease.

There may also be severe lesions, or diseases of the heart, liver or kidneys, which aggravate the condition and make the risk of operation greater than the chance of a successful result. Sometimes a radical operation is out of the question, because the organ concerned is irreplaceable.

But if a surgical operation is not thus precluded, it is often the best solution. According to Bauer, as a "general rule" a decision not to operate should only be taken if the "shortening of life caused by the operation is, all things considered, greater than that due to the cancer".

The "electric knife" causes less haemorrhage

Nowadays the "knife" is no longer the only instrument available for such operations. Elaborate operative techniques, which are constantly being improved, have not completely excluded the risks of surgery, but have at least reduced them. One of these advances is electro-surgery. In this the traditional incision instruments are replaced by cutting electrodes. A relatively large electrode delivers a high-frequency alternating current to the field of operation. The current is then passed to an operating electrode, which is as small as possible. Because the current from the large electrode concentrates into the much smaller operating electrode, very great heat develops there by which the tissue cells are literally "cooked".

This method not only causes less haemorrhage than surgery with the scalpel, but there is also less risk of spreading the cancer cells, since they are completely destroyed and cannot adhere to the operator's knife.

But the electric knife may itself one day be replaced by hollow instruments filled with liquid nitrogen, by ultrasonics or by laser beams. Where nowadays the surgeon spends three-quarters of his time avoiding haemorrhage, these instruments of the future will eliminate the problem completely.

Even the cold probes, hollow needles full of liquid nitrogen, which helped in America to found a new branch of surgery called cryosurgery, seem by comparison with laser beams relatively crude instruments. Cold instruments can be used at temperatures of –20 degrees to –150 degrees C. and can be accurately applied to even a single layer of cells. The hot laser beam, on the other hand, can be concentrated on tissues with the incredible accuracy of fractions of one thousandth of a millimetre in diameter.

Dr. Irving S. Cooper of the New York St. Barnabas Hospital, at 42 years of age already one of the pioneers of cryosurgery, predicts a great future for the laser beam in the treatment of cancer. It will, he thinks, acquire a special place in the removal of tumours permeated by numerous blood vessels which tend to form metastases: tumours, that is to say, on which operations are not yet undertaken because of the risk of haemorrhage. Some patients with a very malignant form of skin cancer (Melanoma) have already been treated with the laser beam. The results were positive, though it is still too soon to speak of definite curative results.

Still hotter than the laser beam, hotter even than the surface of the sun, are "plasma jets" – rays of ionised gas – which American doctors are already examining. The physicist Dr. Charles Sheer, of the Electronics Research Laboratory of Columbia University, with the surgeon Robert F. Shaw, conceived the "plasma-arc-scalpel" primarily to permit bloodless operations.

Surgery with the "Jet-cutter"

Plasma is the ionised gas, of which, for example, the luminous surface of the stars is composed. A "plasma jet stream" obtains its energy, not from combustion in the ordinary sense of the term, but from the transformation of electric energy into ions and electrons. This happens when a hot gas is led through an electromagnetic field. The "jet-cutter" should enable surgeons to cut through tissues in a still more simple and more precise way. By contact with this unique scalpel, scientists prophesy, cells will undergo nothing short of evaporation, and those that remain will be cauterised, sterilised and maintained free of haemorrhage.

The infinitely fine needle of the hot plasma stream is surrounded by a coating of cool gas in order to protect the tissues near the operation area.

"Only after this new instrument has proved itself to be absolutely reliable in operations on animals and in selected operations on man, will it be available for general surgery" says Dr. Shaw, and his colleague Sheer continues, "Nothing like the cutting edge of the plasma scalpel has been hitherto available. It is by far the hottest energy ever produced by man, with the possible exception of the fire ball which occurs in an atom bomb explosion."

With laser beams and plasma scalpels the border line between surgical and radiological treatment will diminish still more, as will their areas of use. For example, for many years the treatment for carcinoma of the cervix has been radiology. On the other hand, surgeons have also reported sensational results in treating this form of cancer. In the clinic of the Sloan-Kettering Institute in New York operations have been performed in recent years on 703 patients with carcinoma of the cervix. More than half of them, 57.3 per cent, were still alive five years later; they were cured, according to the usual time limit for cancer. Whilst the survival rate in radiological treatment in the U.S.A. is only slightly above this, the German clinicians led by the University Women's Clinic in Munich show still more impressive results.

The future of radiation treatment

The same rays which cause cancer can also destroy it. In principle the same thing happens in both cases. If rays strike cells in sufficiently high doses, they either change a healthy cell into a malignant one or kill it. Destruction does not always occur instantaneously, but may result from injury and changes in the constituents of the cell which only appear after a certain time has elapsed.

Radioactive irradiation is very energetic and gives off this energy when it strikes the molecule. Changes in a molecule are due to this sudden "energy shock", though the exact mechanism of change is still obscure. Experiments with macromolecules have shown that radiation, for instance, caused cross-linkage compounds in polyvinyl alcohol or split the molecule in haemocyanin. On the other hand, enzymes may be inactivated by radiation.

At present we still do not know what processes are initiated in the complex system of the cell by radiation. Only its effects can be proved without doubt. It has been shown that radiation can cause injuries in all parts of the cell – in both the nucleus and the cytoplasm or in the cell membrane. The nucleoli are just as open to attack as the mitochondria. Moreover, because the nucleus and the cytoplasm mutually influence each other, injuries in the cytoplasm affect the nucleus. The nucleus, however, has proved itself to be relatively more resistant than the cytoplasm when it is irradiated by itself. On the other hand, if nuclei that have not been irradiated are put into irradiated cytoplasm, they also become damaged.

Thus radiation can injure a cell in many ways. For example cell-division may be inhibited, or fractures in the chromosomes can be found. But changes in the DNA of the cell nucleus are the main effect. Among these are modifications of the DNA matrix, inhibition of the synthesis of DNA and splitting up of the DNA and protein complexes. It is significant that such injuries in the cell do not occur immediately, but are observed only after a latent period of time, during which chemical processes, the nature of which is at present still unknown, must have occurred in the cell.

The sensitivity of healthy cells to radiation varies according to the kind of tissue. Cells of the lymphatic system and the bone marrow react the most vigorously. When, for example, the whole body is irradiated with small doses of 5 and 25 Röntgen units, injuries of the lymphocytes can be detected, and with doses of 600 r hardly any undamaged lymphocytes remain 8–10 hours after the application.

In the bone marrow injuries are generally only of consequence if the whole body is irradiated, since the total quantity of this tissue is such the local injuries are not of very serious import. Besides, the bone marrow regenerates itself relatively quickly and well after local irradiation. This is true of doses as high as 9,000 r, when given as a single dose. If, on the other hand, the dose is divided into 30 irradiations, then atrophy of the bone marrow occurs.

The skin reacts even to doses of 350–1,000 r. Temporary loss of hair on the affected places and inhibition of activity of the sweat glands result. After 2,000–3,000 r oedema and pigmentation appear. These are followed, often months or even years later, by atrophy of parts of the epidermis, with speckled pigmentation and reduction of the capillaries. Ulcers may also appear.

Mucous membranes may also react to overdoses of irradiation by the formation of ulcers. This occurs, in some cases, weeks later, but in other cases after the lapse of years or even decades. Doses of 3,000 r cause painful swellings of mucous membranes.

New formation of the epithelial cells of the intestine is decreased by a few hundred r and is stopped by a few thousand r. Irradiation of glands with correspondingly high doses causes temporary or permanent suspension of their activity. In the liver, cirrhosis occurs as a late development. After irradiation with about 2,000 r, shrinkage of the affected parts of the kidney occurs, and may result in cirrhosis of the kidney and uraemia. Irradiation of the tissues of the central nervous system may lead, after a lapse of months, to the formation of cysts. Irradiation of the whole body with extremely high doses of some 10,000 r soon lead to death from damage to the central nervous system.

"X-ray baths" as therapeutic agents

When the destructive effect of X-rays on tumour tissues was discovered, the hope was awakened that the universal therapeutic agent for all kinds of cancer had at last been found. In 1905 the suggestion was made, with unhesitating enthusiasm, of exposing cancer patients to radical irradiation of the whole body. Such an "X-ray bath" would then cure both the primary tumour and also any possible metastases.

But it was soon necessary to accept that things were unfortunately not so simple. As the frequent occurrence of cancerous tumours after intensive or repeated X-ray irradiation showed, radiation damaged not only the tumour cells, as was first thought, but also the healthy tissues.

Thus radiotherapy had to discover how to expose the tumour to active and concentrated radiation as possible, but at the same time to spare the healthy tissues. The continual development of new apparatus and of better methods of irradiation had only one purpose, the concentration of a high dose of radiation on to the cancerous centre while causing as little damage as possible to the rest of the tissues.

Thus radiotherapy, like surgery, can only achieve an effect

where there is a circumscribed tumour. But it can often also be effective in cases where a surgical operation is out of the question because important organs are diseased.

Tumour cells are more vulnerable

In doing this, radiotherapy takes advantage of the fact that many kinds of tumour are more sensitive to the effects of radiation than healthy tissues. The more intensive the divisions of a cell and the less differentiated it is, the more sensitive it becomes. Because it is characteristic of many cancer cells that they are more prone to division, and at the same time more undifferentiated, than normal cells, the effect on them of radiation is generally stronger.

It is true that degrees of sensitivity to radiation are very different in various kinds of tumours.

Lymphosarcomas are especially sensitive, as are tumours of the testes, granulomatous cell tumours and basal cell carcinomas. On the other hand, almost all adenocarcinomas and most sarcomas and brain tumours can be regarded as resistant to radiation.

The American radiological specialist Shields L. Warren divides tumours into three large groups, according to their sensitivity to radiation. The first group includes tumours that undergo involution under irradiation up to a total dose of 2,500 r. Among these Warren places lymphomas, chronic leukaemias and the Ewing-sarcoma of bone. The second group, which includes basal cell carcinomas of the skin, carcinoma of the cervix and adenocarcinomas of the thyroid, requires total doses of 2,500–5,000 r. The third group, which includes carcinomas of the stomach and breast, malignant melanoma and sarcoma of bone, requires more than 5,000 r.

Surprising in this enumeration is the reference to chronic leukaemias, which are not solid tumours. Occasionally in these diseases the whole body has been irradiated. However, there are in this treatment very narrow limits; only minimal doses can be used, for otherwise severe generalised injuries can occur. However, with irradiation of the spleen, in which the white blood corpuscles are formed, encouraging results have already been obtained in chronic leukaemia.

Treatment with fast electrons

When German and French scientists introduced radiological treatment into cancer therapy in the twenties, X-ray equipment was exclusively used. It soon turned out that several thousand radiation units (r or rad) was necessary for the successful treatment of tumours. This is simplest with tumours that lie close under the skin, for here the source of the rays can be brought near to, or even into immediate contact with, the tumour.

More difficult are the much commoner cases in which the tumour is hidden in the interior of the body. In these cases the total required dosage of several thousand rad must be concentrated on the site of the disease, but at the same time the healthy tissue in its neighbourhood must be spared as much as possible. In the course of time, therefore, various methods of irradiation were developed to avoid too much damage to the healthy tissues.

This was achieved by spreading the treatment over several weeks and by a corresponding reduction of each individual dose. In this treatment "by instalments" each irradiation may last only a few minutes.

"Cross-fire" on the tumour

Moreover individual irradiations of a tumour of this kind are applied in variable directions. By this cross-fire treatment, the radiation dose on healthy tissues is reduced to a tolerable level.

Another method is irradiation through a sieve. In this a heavy metal sieve is used which is always placed in the same position on the part of the skin irradiated. In this way the epithelial tissue is only affected at places where the openings in the sieve lie. Elsewhere the rays cannot penetrate the heavy metal.

Then, after the treatment, the damaged areas can easily be regenerated from those that are protected and undamaged. With this method the dose of radiation immediately under the skin is naturally distributed unequally, but the deeper the rays penetrate the more the inequalities even out. The procedure thus protects the skin and makes higher doses of radiation possible.

Despite all these precautionary measures, inflammation of the skin cannot be avoided. Three or four weeks after the commencement of irradiation, symptoms appear which often resemble severe sunburn; but these usually heal in a few weeks.

Even less drastic is the modern high voltage treatment. This is treatment with fast electrons and electro-magnetic wave irradiation. While conventional X-ray tubes work at about 200,000 volts, currents of more than 3 million volts are necessary for ultra-hard Röntgen rays. In deep irradiation the X-ray tube has nowadays been largely superseded by high voltage apparatus.

Such "ultra-hard" Röntgen and gamma rays have considerable advantages over the rays formerly used. They penetrate the material much more intensively, with the result that deep tumours receive a higher dose of radiation. In addition, if rays strike a substance secondary rays develop. With conventional X-rays these secondary rays go in all directions, but with ultra-hard radiation they proceed parallel to the primary radiation, concentrating much more effectively on the site of the disease. Because of this better concentration of the secondary rays the effect of the dose increases and, because ultra-hard radiation is much less damaging to the skin, higher doses can be used.

The Betatron offers a choice of rays

The Gammatron and Betatron are also used to produce powerful rays of this kind. In the Gammatron the source of radiation is a radioactive substance which emits gamma rays as it disintegrates. The radioactivity must amount to several thousand Curies. The element most often used nowadays is Cobalt 60. Such radioactive elements can be supplied by atomic reactors, not only in sufficient quantities but also at reasonable prices. This treatment is therefore gaining ground steadily.

The Betatron – most of those used in Germany provide energies of 15–20 million electron volts – provides fast electrons which can be used for the generation of ultra-hard Röntgen radiation. In the Betatron, electrons are accelerated almost to the speed of light by a magnetic field in a ring-shaped high vacuum tube. The electrons can then be directed outwards and used for clinical irradiation.

At first, such Betatrons, the working principle of which was registered as a patent in 1921 by an American scientist, were required only for physical research. Ten years later the situation changed. Professor Boris Rajewsky in Frankfurt-am-Main, recognised that the electrons alter the enzyme system by chemical reactions when they enter the cell, and thus destroy it. It was ultimately also thanks to Rajewsky that the firm of Siemens-Reiniger undertook the serial production of a Betatron of 42 MeV for medical purposes.

This apparatus is, however, extremely expensive, costing more than £100,000. Obviously a small hospital can hardly afford such an expense, so larger treatment centres must be established which can bear the very high costs.

Apparatus with energies of many millions of electron volts, as well as radioactive cobalt sources, have substantially improved the radiation treatment of tumours. Before their appearance it was only possible to apply 10–15 per cent of the radiation necessary before the treatment had to be broken off because the patient could not tolerate it.

A hard-ray bunker in Giessen

Nowadays the whole necessary dose can almost always be applied, explains Professor Gunther Barth, Director of the Giessen X-ray clinic. This clinic possesses the most modern radiation equipment. In a "hard-ray bunker" in the grounds of the University of Giessen there is an 18-million electron volt Betatron, a Gammatron and a radiocobalt source with a radiation strength of 400 Curies. The treatment rooms lie deep under the earth and are surrounded by thick concrete walls. The building costs of the bunker alone were nearly £250,000. This expensive installation guarantees the protection of medical and service personnel from the effects of radiation.

However, attempts to improve the prospects of radiotherapy are not only made by the use of hard rays. New methods of application which allow better protection of healthy tissues, also help to do this. These include moving or rotating irradiation, in which the source of the radiation rotates along segments of a circle of which the tumour is the centre. In this way the centre of disease in the interior of the body receives the highest possible dose of radiation, while the healthy layers of tissue traversed by the rays on their way to the tumour are varied. This tissue is thus less damaged than it would be if subjected to constant irradiation from the same direction. In this way much higher doses can be used.

Cancer therapy may perhaps have recourse in the future, in addition to fast electrons, to other corpuscular rays, such as neutrons and protons. Neutron rays would have the advantage that their effect is not dependent on the presence of oxygen. In past research, however, delayed injuries to the skin have often resulted from this treatment.

The other promising possibility would be treatment with protons, for considerable technical difficulties have initially to be overcome. In the use of protons, which can attain a very high ionisation in a limited space, it is first necessary to have an extensive proton accelerator. In addition it is necessary to work with very high energies; to produce rays which penetrate into the middle of the body about 170 MeV are absolutely necessary. The voltage of the apparatus, moreover, cannot be varied, so that one would have to use these energies in all cases.

Finally, attempts are still being made to increase the efficiency of radiation therapy by additional devices. In any event malignant cells seem to react more vigorously than healthy cells, but the sensitivity of tumours can be increased still further in many cases by certain chemicals or by a change in the gas-atmosphere. A chemical compound which, according to Dr. R. Schindler of Lausanne, sensitizes cells to irradiation is 5-Bromdesoxyuridin. It is incorporated by the cell into the DNA.

Professor I. Churchill-Davidson calls attention to another possibility. He starts from the fact that deprivation of oxygen – for example, irradiation in nitrogen – protects cells to a large extent from radiation injury. He assumes that most tumours contain a small percentage of cells that are deficient in oxygen. They would thus be resistant to radiation and a new tumour could develop from them. But an increased supply of oxygen during irradiation must make these cells, too, susceptible to radiation. In fact, research in London has shown that patients irradiated under high oxygen pressure survive much better than those treated in normal air, and that there are fewer relapses among them.

Visit to the Radiumhemmet

Dr. Gustaf Notter, too, hopes for considerable advances in cancer radiotherapy from the further development of such combined methods. "This kind of treatment will certainly increase in importance," says Dr. Notter, provisional director of the Radiumhemmet in Stockholm, the oldest radiation clinic in Europe.

The Radiumhemmet, founded in 1910, owes its existence to the initiative of Professor John Berg, who pioneered cancer control in Sweden and ultimately, with two friends, collected the sum of 40,000 crowns to set up a private radiation clinic in a Stockholm block of flats.

The clinic began with an X-ray unit, 120 milligrams of radium, and 16 beds for in-patient treatment. Today it has more than 150 beds and a total staff of 22 doctors in its general and gynaecological departments. Its equipment is extremely modern. It includes, in addition to installations for classical X-ray treatment, about 10 grams of radium, several cobalt sources, including sources that supply 2,500 and 6,000 Curies, as well as a Betatron of 17 MeV. Another Betatron of 42 MeV will soon be installed.

The Radiumhemmet is no longer a private organisation. It belongs to the Karolinska Institutet, the famous medical school of Stockholm, which awards the Nobel Prize for medicine every year. The costs are borne by the Swedish State, from the Jubilee Fund of King Gustaf V., by the Stockholm Cancer Society and various other associations and organisations.

The clinic confines itself exclusively to radiotherapy and directly associated research. But it is closely connected with two other radiological Institutes of the Medical School. One is the Institute for Radiophysics, concerned with all problems of radiophysics and particularly with anti-radiation precautions. Among these are the supervision of X-ray equipment and the evaluation of records from the 37 metering stations belonging to the institute, which test the radioactive content of the atmosphere in the various parts of Sweden.

Separate diagnosis and treatment

The second of these institutes, the Institute of Radiopathology, is concerned with tissue cultures, tissue research and diagnosis. This separation of diagnosis in the Radiopathology Institute from actual treatment in the Radiumhemmet is regarded in Stockholm as extremely important. "This separation does not yet exist in most other European countries, in France, Italy and the Federal Republic of Germany," says Dr. Notter. "This is because in these countries the special position of radiotherapists is still not acknowledged to the degree it is by us. In these countries, radiologists would scarcely be understood if they claimed a further subdivision of their responsibility. But we are convinced that such limitation and specialisation is absolutely necessary, and that our system of separating diagnosis from treatment will succeed in the long run."

This is only one example of the complex co-operation of different specialists. It is characteristic not only in the radiological approach to cancer, but also in its general treatment. The results are groupings such as the Radiumhemmet and its sister institutes of the Stockholm Medical School. The exchange of experience and of the results of research and treatment is guaranteed. But the individual specialist can devote his undivided attention to his own sphere of work, and can develop such new methods of treatment as the combination of radiation and oxygen.

Oxygen and cancer cells

Cancer cells can be saturated with oxygen in different ways. For example, hydrogen peroxide can be led through a catheter into the arteries which directly supply the tumour region. This method has been already perfected in a clinic in Dallas, Texas. The patient can also be exposed to an increase of oxygen in a pressure chamber. When this is done, an overpressure of up to three atmospheres can be used. Still higher pressure may cause convulsions which necessitate narcosis before treatment.

When the overpressure method is used, it could be expected that the oxygen saturation of all cells would occur. In practice, the oxygen content of the normal cells increases only slightly, whereas that of the cancer cells increases substantially, thereby rendering them more sensitive to radiation. One per cent of malignant cells, which without oxygen would survive an irradiation, would be enough for the formation of a new tumour.

At present it is still almost impossible to detect an increased oxygen content in human tumour cells, for the methods of measuring it are still too crude. Because this treatment leads to better results, however, a stronger saturation of cancer cells with oxygen may be inferred.

Not only may the oxygen content of malignant cells be increased, but it is also possible to lower it in the surrounding healthy cells. This method is mainly used in the treatment of limbs or the lobes of the lungs.

Mice in the low-pressure chamber

Whilst radiotherapy is going on together with over-pressure treatment in the Radiumhemmet, members of another institute in Stockholm University, the Radiobiological Institute, are working in the opposite direction. In this institute Dr. Bernhard Tribukait exposes mice to low pressure and then irradiates them.

Male mice of an internationally recognised breeding stock were first kept for 10 days in a low-pressure chamber. The pressure corresponded to that of an altitude of 6,000 metres. This caused a lack of oxygen (hypoxia) in the tissues. Then Tribukait irradiated the mice with total doses of 750–1,350 r. This was done at different times, varying from immediately after their sojourn in the low-pressure chamber to 1–4 days later. In comparison with control mice living under normal oxygen conditions, these showed interesting changes in their sensitivity to irradiation. The results of irradiation with a total dose of about 1,000 r derived from a cobalt source were especially interesting. The death rate among the mice suffering from hypoxia was considerably lower than that among the control mice. Of the mice not treated, 72.5 per cent died within 30 days of irradiation. In the same periods between 22.8 per cent and 52.6 per cent of the mice with hypoxia died, depending on the interval between the hypoxia and the irradiation.

But there was still another phenomenon. Among the mice which were not exposed to low-pressure, death occurred mainly on the 11th–12th day after the irradiation. None died before the 10th day. But among the mice irradiated a few minutes after the hypoxia, early deaths were recorded even between the 5th and 8th day.

This happened in about 25 per cent of these mice, but the total number of survivors after 30 days was still higher than that among the control mice.

Early deaths decreased considerably if irradiation was given one, two or three days after hypoxia. Simultaneously the number of survivors increased markedly. With irradiation after four days the total number of deaths again increased.

Dr. Tribukait concluded from these results that an increased sensitivity to irradiation develops immediately after the hypoxia, but that this is then succeeded in subsequent days by increased resistance to irradiation. Ultimately the sensitivity to irradiation becomes the same as that of untreated animals.

Further experiments were conducted to determine the consequences of irradiation during the first 24 hours after hypoxia. The animals were irradiated 5 minutes, and 3, 6, 15 and 24 hours after hypoxia. The number of deaths from irradiation 3, 6 and 15 hours after hypoxia was much greater than it was in control animals. Moreover, most of the animals died more quickly. With an irradiation six hours after hypoxia, for example, all the animals died within 17 days, and few survived the 10th day. With irradiation 24 hours after hypoxia there were hardly any early deaths. After 30 days, 34.3 per cent of the animals survived as against only 13.6 per cent among the controls.

What causes the changes in sensitivity to irradiation after hypoxia? The research workers in Stockholm have not yet been able to answer this question. Still, these experiments could ultimately provide knowledge valuable to radiation biology and perhaps lead eventually to new treatments.

Destruction of tumours from within

Professor Dr. Lee F. Farr of the American cancer research centre in Brookhaven also reports on a new method of irradiation. In Farr's researches, which have still not progressed beyond the stage of experiments on animals, a boron compound, sodium pentaborate, is injected intravenously. This compound has two noteworthy characteristics. It collects preferentially in cancer cells, and also absorbs neutrons very well. If the cancerous tumour is now attacked with a stream of neutrons, the boron present is converted into radioactive Lithium 7, which decays by emitting alpha particles. However, its range of action is not very great.

By this means it might be possible to destroy the tumour from within, without damaging the surrounding tissues too much. However, one would certainly encounter difficulties which occur in every radiation treatment of larger tumours. When, for example large cell populations are destroyed, toxic protein decomposition products are set free and these may lead to very unpleasant side-effects – in extreme cases, to uraemia. Thus there seem to be certain limits to successful treatment.

There are good chances for the radiotherapy of tumours which the surgeon can expose but cannot remove, for such tumours can be irradiated directly. Usually, as Professor Barth of Giessen reported, a dose sufficient to destroy the tumour can then be given to almost all patients.

Malignant tumours can be caused by physical influences, for example, by irradiation, chemical substances (such as benzpyrene), and by viruses, for example, the Rous sarcoma virus of chickens.

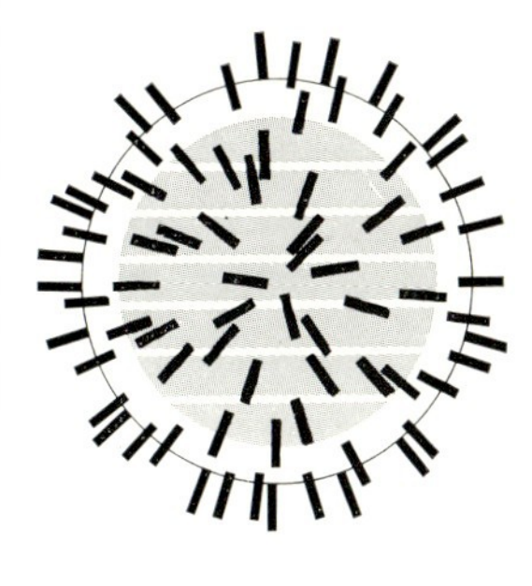

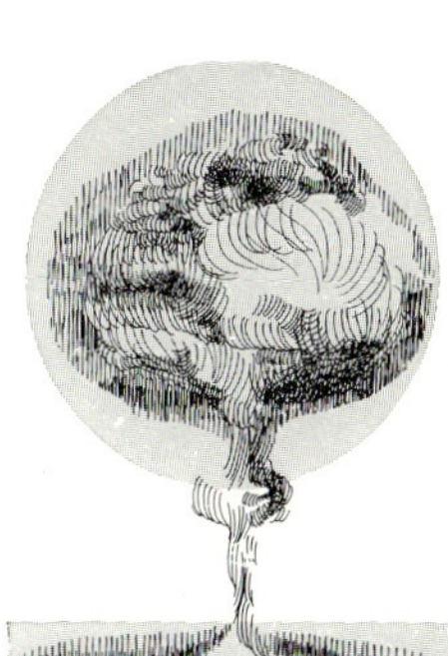

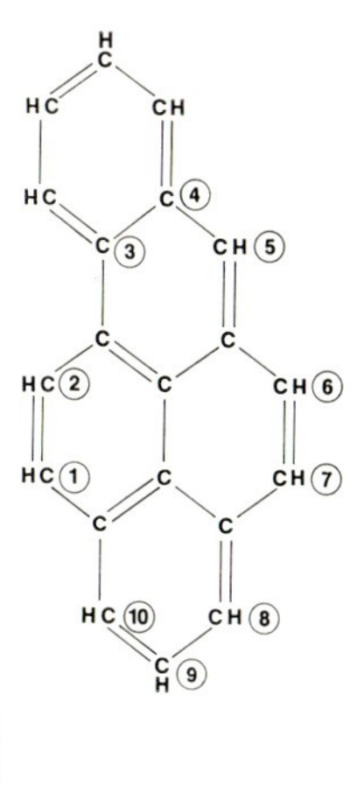

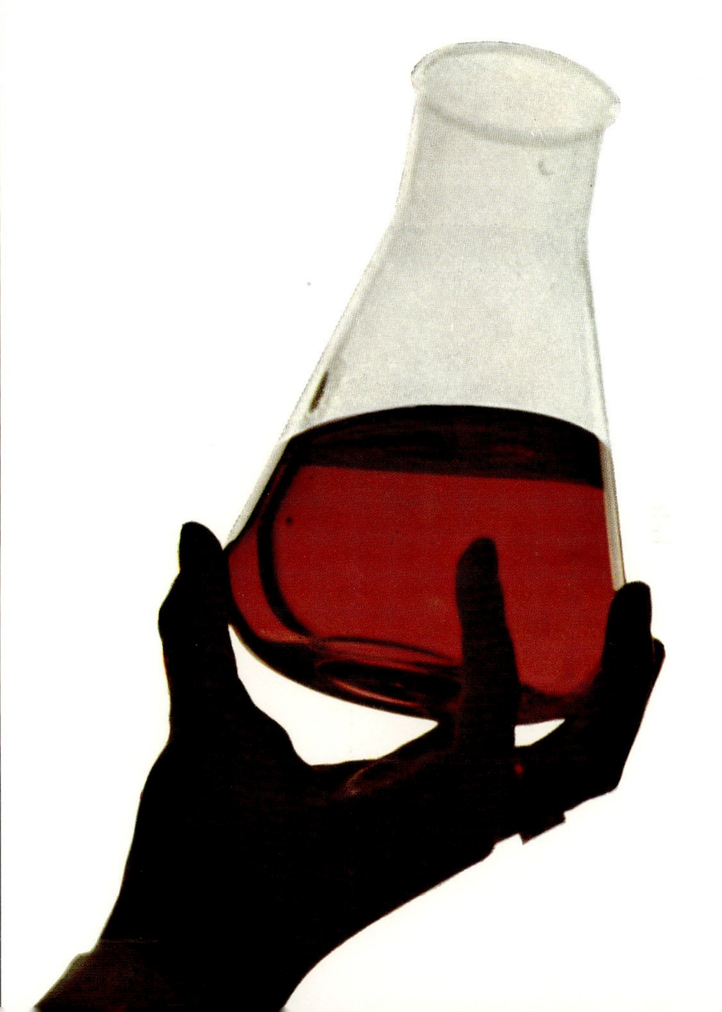

Thanks to the initiative of Professor Karl Heinrich Bauer, the German Cancer Research Centre was established in Heidelberg.
Our picture shows the first stages in its development. Fundamental research will be undertaken here.

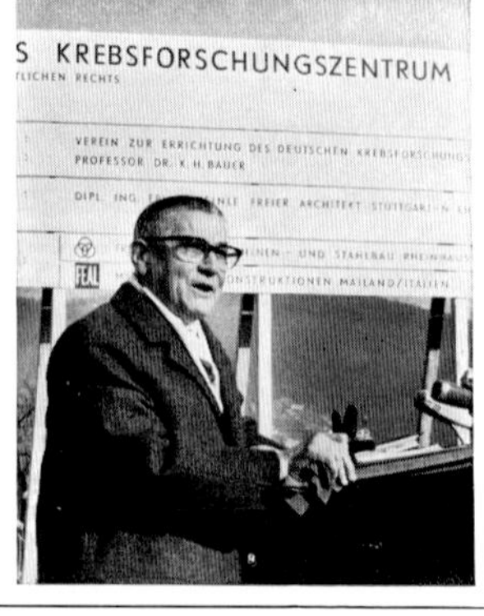

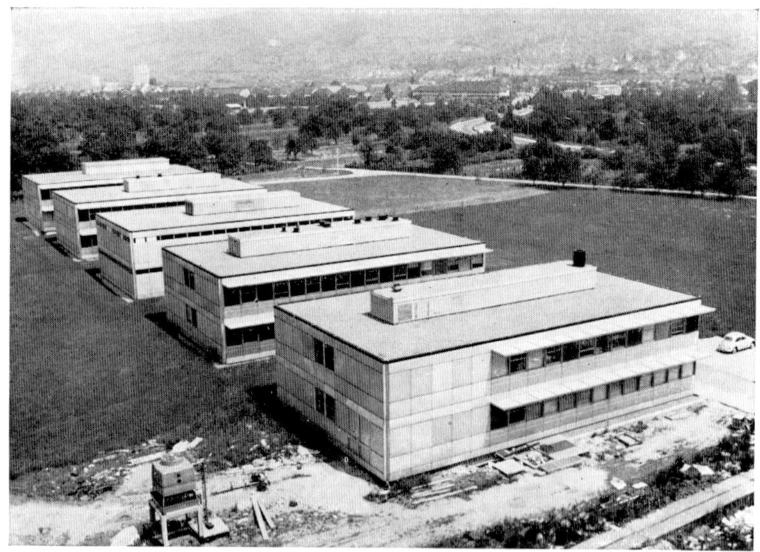

The penetration of virus-nucleic acid into the cell decides its fate. Our diagram shows this proccss. The coloured photograph represents a tumour caused by a virus—the Rous sarcoma described by the American Nobel Prize Laureate Peyton-Rous.

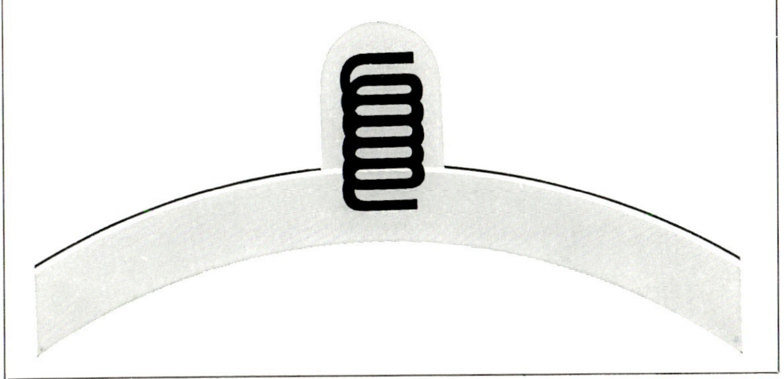

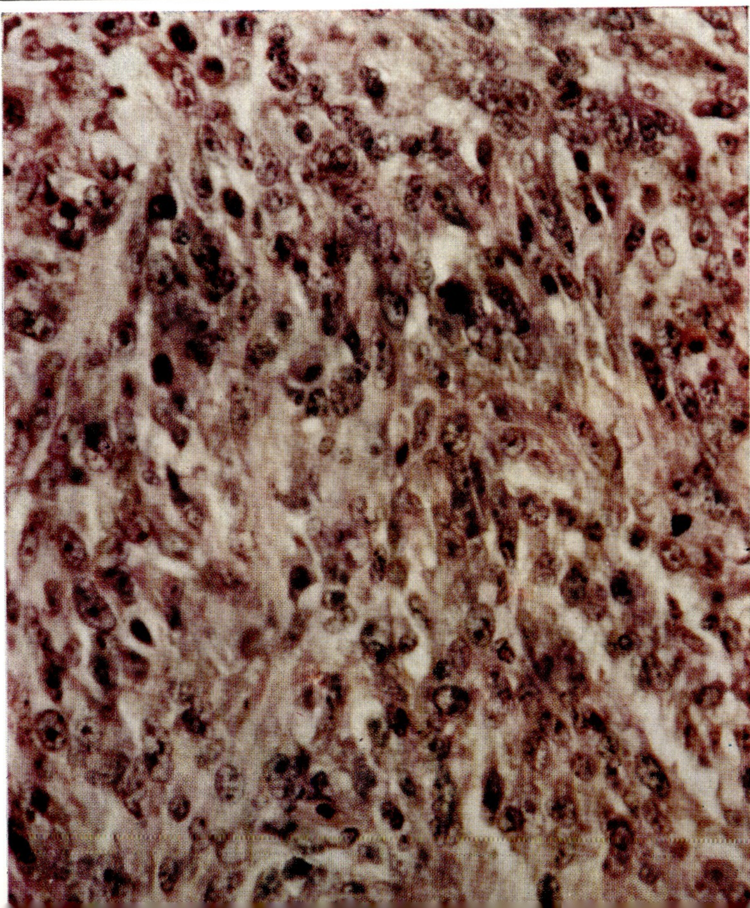

A partial view of a stronghold of cancer research, the Sloan Kettering Institute in New York.

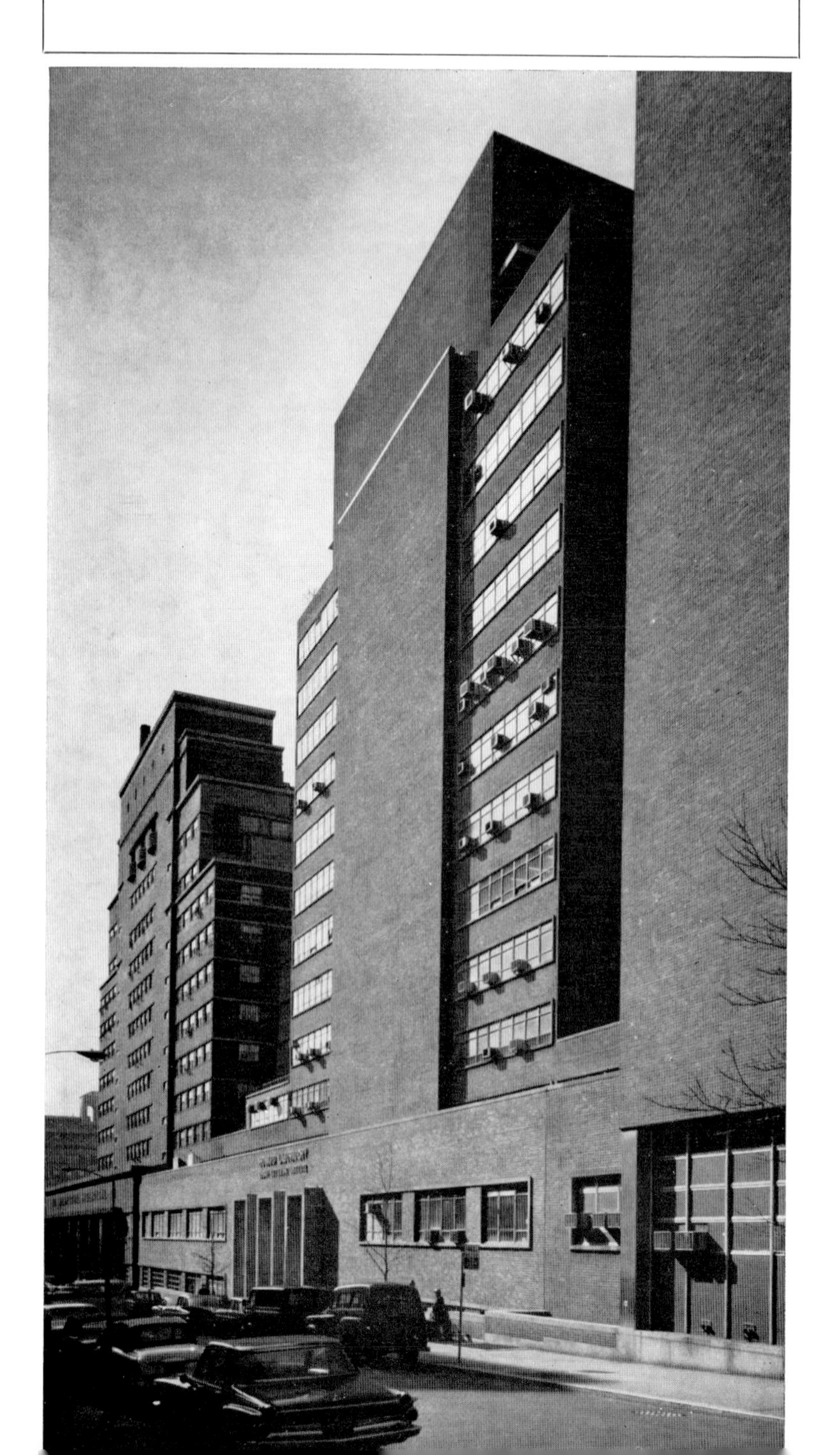

Ludvik Gross was the first to prove that a leukaemia in mice is caused by a virus. In the electron microscope photograph the viruses appear in various places as dark circular structures.

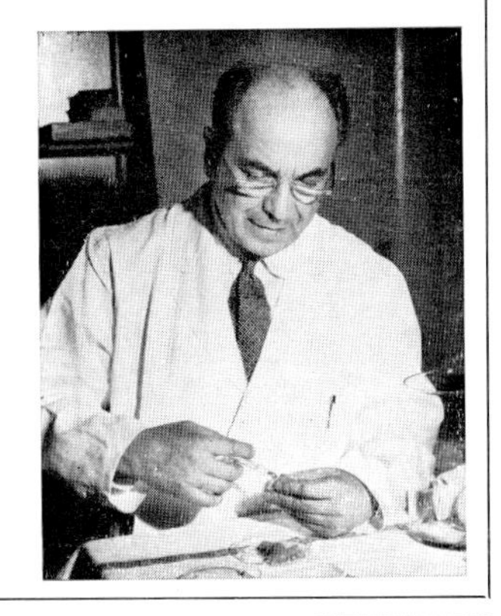

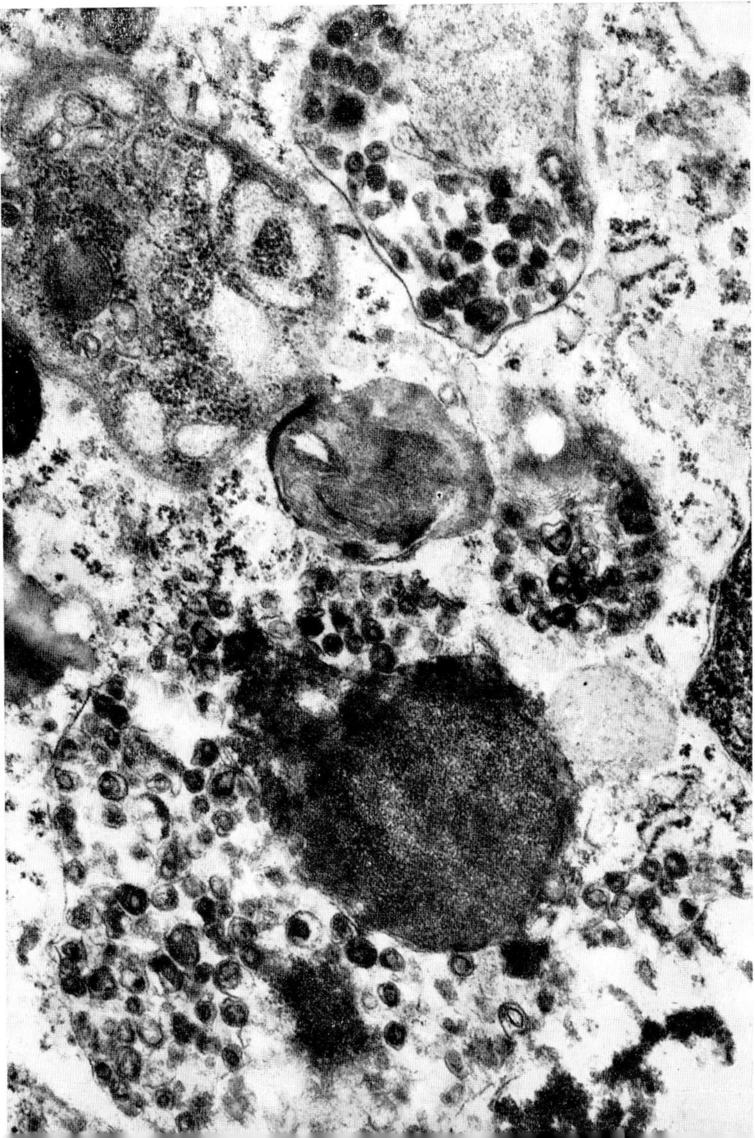

The two American virologists, Dr. Sarah Stewart (top) and Dr. Bernice Eddy (bottom)are world-famous. They discovered the oncogenic features of the polyoma virus. They work in the National Institutes of Health at Bethesda, near Washington.

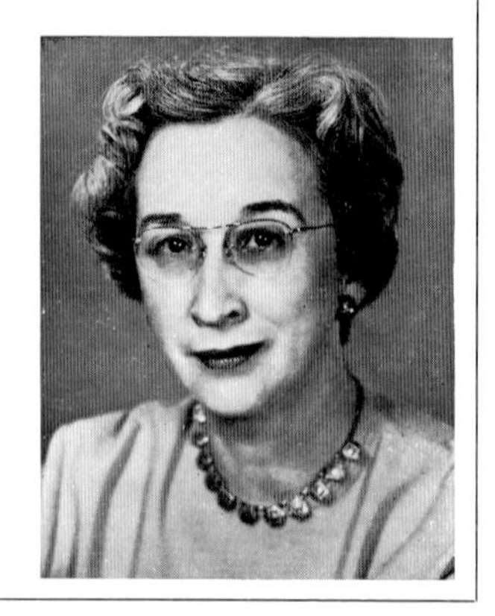

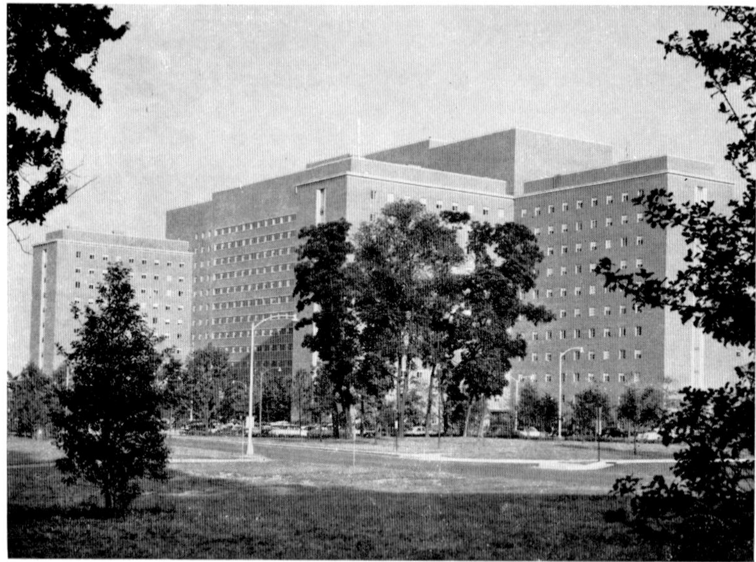

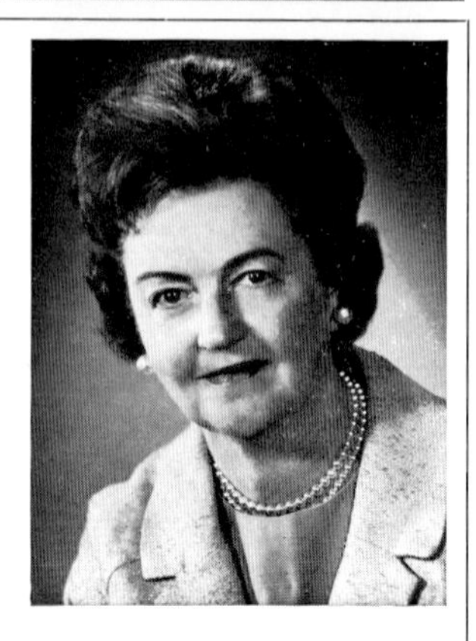

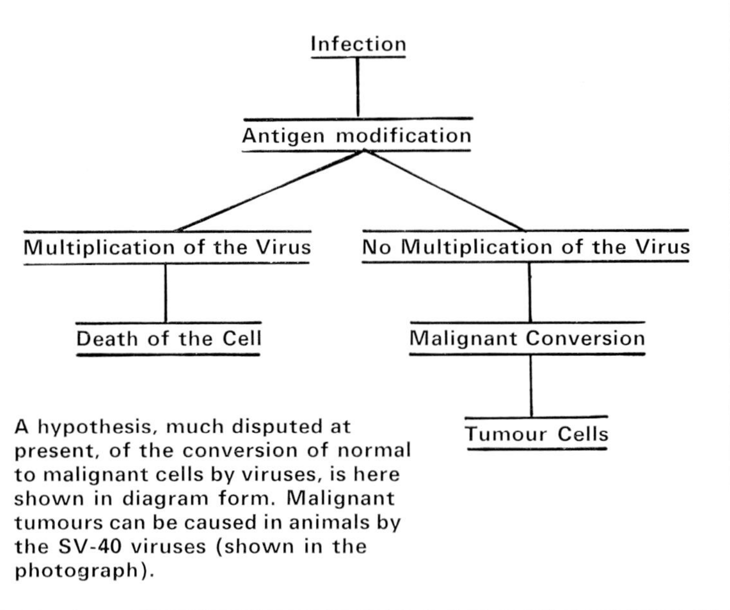

A hypothesis, much disputed at present, of the conversion of normal to malignant cells by viruses, is here shown in diagram form. Malignant tumours can be caused in animals by the SV-40 viruses (shown in the photograph).

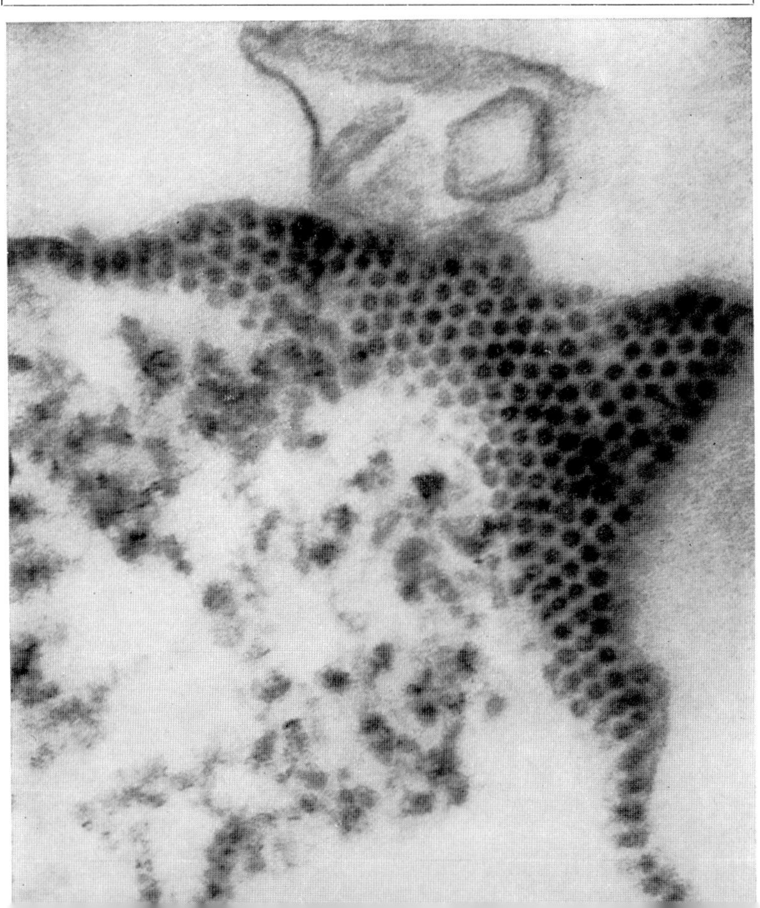

Adeno-viruses under the electron microscope. Some members of this group of viruses cause the formation of tumours in Golden hamsters.

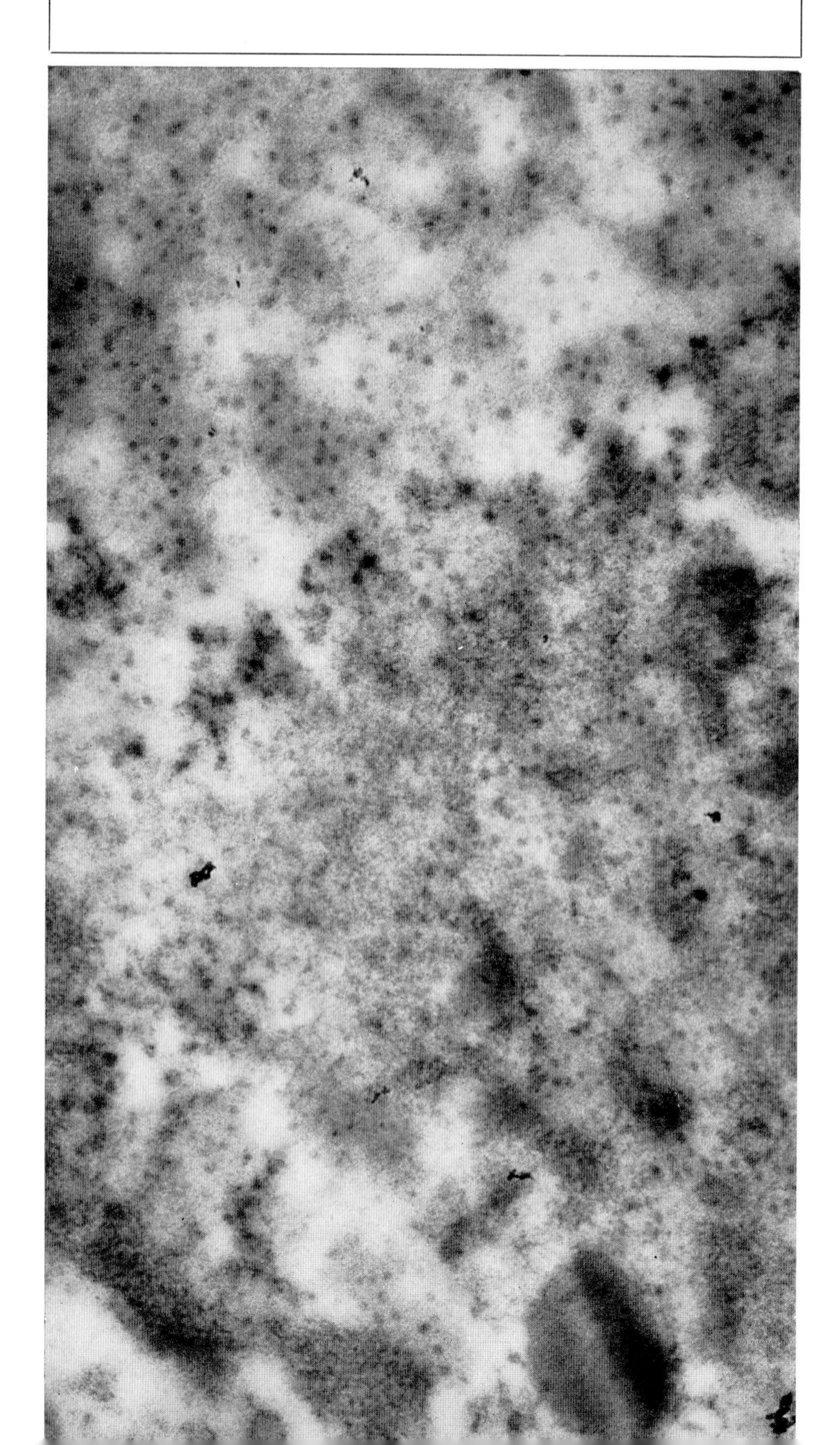

Ultra-hard rays have considerably improved the chances of successful treatment in comparison with conventional irradiation. Professor Werner Hellriegel, Director of the Radiological Clinic in the Bürger-Katharinen Hospital in Stuttgart has produced comparative figures. In the X-ray treatment of lymphosarcomas and reticulosarcomas 23 per cent of the patients were alive after three years and 12 per cent after five years. On the other hand, of another group of patients with sarcomas of the same origin and in comparable stages of development, 33 per cent were alive after three years and 23 per cent after five years following treatment with ultra-hard rays.

Hellriegel obtained similar results with carcinoma of the larynx in the first and second stage of the disease. With X-ray treatment the survival rate after five years amounted to 45 per cent of the patients, but to 60 per cent with electron radiation.

Another example is the treatment of cancer of the mammary glands in the first and second stages of development. If this is first operated upon and then treated with X-rays, the chance of survival after four years amounts to 57 per cent. If the X-ray treatment is given before the operation, this survival rate increases to 72 per cent. But, if the operation is preceded by irradiation with fast electrons the survival rate after four years reaches 80 per cent. In the third and fourth stage also, when metastases are already present, the use of ultra-hard radiation improves the chance of survival by 20 per cent.

In carcinoma of the cervix surgical operation, like irradiation – here combined with additional deposits of radium – both have their place. In tumours in the digestive tract on the other hand, i.e. in the intestine, stomach, gall bladder and the pancreas, an operation is almost always preferred. With brain tumours, tumours of the breast, the ovary and of the limbs and muscles, too, the surgeon generally has the first word. Often the surgeon and radiologist work hand in hand, since irradiation before and after operations reduces the risk of the formation of metastases by the dissemination of malignant cells.

Radio-isotopes and the tumour

In addition to methods of irradiation in which the source of the rays is brought to the body from the outside, there are also methods by which the irradiation is applied internally by means of radioactive isotopes. Such isotopes include, for example, those of phosphorus, cobalt, iodine and gold.

An important characteristic of the radio-isotope is its half-life, i.e. the period of time taken for half of the material to disintegrate. This half-life differs greatly among the individual isotopes. That of radioactive cobalt 60 is 5.2 years; that of radioactive gold 198, on the other hand, is only 2.7 days. Naturally the thought occurs of using such radio-isotopes for treatment, and in many cases this has already been done. If a way can be found of bringing the radioactive material directly into the tumour, the tumour will be destroyed from within. The surrounding healthy tissue can be better protected than when irradiation is applied externally.

One possible method of using radioactive isotopes is by their application to body cavities. If the radioactive substance is enclosed in small tubes, capsules or plasticine, it can be brought via these cavities directly to the tumour, i.e. into the nose and throat, abdominal cavity or bladder. It can also be implanted in the brain in artificial cavities created by the surgeon. Another possibility is to embed the radio-isotope directly into the tumour. This can also be done in the form of solutions or suspensions, in which instance the body excretes the isotope after some time.

Some elements are stored up in certain tissues or organs of the body. If a radioactive isotope of such an element is put into the body, it accumulates in the specific tissue. In bones, for example, phosphorus 32, strontium 40 and yttrium 90 accumulate; the liver attracts cobalt 60 and gold 198, and the thyroid, iodine 131.

This is a decided advantage in the treatment of cancer of the thyroid. First, radioactive iodine is given to the patient as a "detector substance". It concentrates not only in the thyroid gland, but also in the cancer cells that have already migrated to other parts of the body. Instruments of the Geiger counter type can determine where the foci of cancer have been formed. Then the thyroid gland is surgically removed, and the patient is given a radioactive "iodine cocktail" to drink. Its radiation then affects the other cancer cells which have separated from the thyroid gland.

But not all cases of cancer of the thyroid can be treated in this way. The reason for this is that cancer cells, as has already been mentioned, often lose their differentiation. In this way tumour tissue often loses the specific features of the original organ, in this instance, the thyroid, and simultaneously loses the ability to store iodine. The tumour will therefore only respond to radio-isotopes while the cancer cells are still relatively differentiated.

Finally, malignant diseases of the blood are also treated with radio-isotopes, especially with phosphorus 32. For these the preparation is given either orally or intravenously. But the radioactive substance acts not only on the malignant but also on the normal blood and body cells, so there are also strict limits to this treatment.

Chemical weapons against cancer

Treatment by surgery or irradiation are both powerless if the tumour has, by the time it is first diagnosed and treated, formed secondary tumours in widely separated parts of the body. In such instances help can only be given by chemical weapons which can kill cancer cells wherever they may be found in the body. In 1889 Theodor Billroth, one of the great surgeons, said: "Chemistry must provide the desired solution, for, in cancer, our art and skill all too often fail."

Preparations effective against any kind of tumour cells in any part of the body would spell victory over cancer. To millions of people devoted to science it seems inconceivable that, in an era of supersonic aeroplanes and space rockets, such a compound has not been found. Have not research workers eradicated infectious diseases in industrialised countries with the help of antibiotics? In understandable impatience people all over the world await the headline: "Cancer cure discovered."

But when will it actually come? Or, to put it in another way: will there ever be a remedy that destroys all forms of cancer? No scientist can today forecast this, although all over the world gigantic efforts are being made. In America especially attempts – supported both nationally and privately – are being made to master the cancer problem chemotherapeutically.

The efforts and the financial expenditure involved are among the greatest in the history of civilisation. They exceed even those of the atom bomb. In a matchless test programme American scientists screen every new chemical compound, vegetable substances from all parts of the earth, soil fungi and hormones, for their possible effects on cancer. In the privately financed Sloan-Kettering Institute in New York, which plays a leading part in chemotherapy, 100,000 substances have so far been tested for their effect on cancer.

Hardly any investigator believes in the discovery of a preparation that would overcome all forms of cancer alike. In hundreds of laboratories men would consider themselves lucky to find a preparation that would cure even one of the commonest forms of cancer. For chemical substances have so far brought only partial success – they can reduce the tumour and give people suffering from cancer a reprieve of weeks, months and sometimes even years.

The price, for the most part, is high. There are almost always quite considerable side-effects. Still, the last 10 or 15 years have brought a considerable advance in chemotherapy. The span of life is increased, the spectrum of efficiency is broader and the side-effects are fewer. A genuine cure has even been reported of a comparatively rare form of cancer – tumours of the placenta.

The great hope is chemotherapy

But when will there be cures of lung cancer or tumours of the digestive tract by means of chemical "magic bullets"? Only with their help will it be possible to achieve in the future a further drastic reduction of death rates, for the classical methods of combating cancer have without doubt reached the limit of their potentiality. As Dr Werner von Droste of the surgical clinic of the University of Heidelberg sums it up in his broad essay, 'Results of 25 years of combating cancer by clinical surgery': "We have arrived at a stage when, in the battle against cancer, our existing weapons produce good results, but have come to a definite standstill."

The President of the American Cancer Society, Dr. Wendell Scott, has expressed himself recently no less clearly; "The existing techniques of both surgery and irradiation, either alone or in combination, have attained their maximal effect in the treatment of human cancer." All hopes are therefore now centred on chemotherapy.

Chapter 6

IN THE WORKSHOP OF THE CHEMOTHERAPISTS

Bari, the Italian seaport on the Adriatic, comes into the history of cancer therapy thanks to the Allied Bomber Force. In 1944, war planes attacked freighters in the harbour and hit a storeroom which contained large quantities of mustard gas – a dreaded war gas of the First World War called Sulphur Mustard.

Many people inhaled this poisonous compound and became severely ill: and doctors found in them a drastic reduction of the number of white blood corpuscles and grave injury to the bone marrow, in which the leucocytes are produced. These were changes very similar to those which may also appear in people exposed to very high doses of radiation.

Possibly this incident would have remained completely unnoticed in the confusion of the last years of the war, if there had not been among the Allied staff some scientists who saw that this gas had more than a military interest. Thus, in Great Britain, Eric Boyland and, in particular, Charlotte Auerbach were able to prove, for the first time, that sulphur mustard could cause mutations.

Soon chemists and doctors had discovered how this substance causes death: it destroys the blood-forming tissue. In this way the marked reduction of leucocytes also occurred. Nitrogen mustard in which the sulphur atom is replaced by nitrogen, also has this property.

Nobody would previously have contemplated the introduction of such a poisonous substance into cancer therapy. But leukaemia acts by flooding the blood with immature white blood corpuscles, and therefore the idea arose of using sulphur mustard against leukaemia. Until then surgery could not do much against this form of cancer, and irradiation also had little effect.

Still during the war, Dr. Alfred Gilman of the Medical School of Harvard began to study the pharmacological properties of mustard gas and to treat the first patients. All these researches had to be done in strict secrecy, but in 1946 Dr. Cornelius Packard Rhoads, Head of the Memorial Cancer Hospital in New York, reported on clinical experiences in the treatment of 160 patients suffering from leukaemia and lymphomata.

In almost all these cases astonishing improvements were recorded, especially in the so-called Hodgkin's disease (lymphogranulomatosis), a tumour-like disease which primarily attacks the lymph glands and was first described in 1832 by the English doctor Thomas Hodgkin. It chiefly affects young people 20–30 years old.

Naturally this treatment was very risky. After all, nitrogen-mustard was an extremely poisonous compound, originally intended not for the salvation of human life, but for its destruction. However carefully these early cases were dosed, injuries to the blood forming organs were almost always recorded.

It was therefore necessary to remodel these compounds in such a way that they remained completely effective but were decisively diminished in toxicity. Chemical substances were needed, the injurious effect of which would be maximal on cancer cells, but minimal on healthy cells. Alexander Haddow and his colleagues of the Chester Beatty Institute in London, searching for less toxic nitrogen-mustard derivatives, developed the compound chlorambucil, or leukeran. It can be used successfully against chronic lymphatic leukaemia, but also against other forms of blood-cancer and lymphomata. Blood-formation is only slightly inhibited by this compound, though this effect cannot be reversed.

When chlorine atoms are split off

The purely clinical results of this work at the Chester Beatty Institute were just as important in another way. In the course of this work the properties of the nitrogen mustard derivatives, which were responsible for the growth-inhibiting effects of these compounds, were discovered. It was shown that the chlorine atoms contained in all mustard gas preparations almost certainly play the chief part. When, for example, nitrogen mustard is injected and is dissolved in the body fluids, hydrochloric acid is split off and the rest of the preparation combines with various molecules inside the cell, including the proteins and nucleic acids. But a direct combination of nitrogen mustard with proteins is also possible. This process is called alkylation.

Chemically very different substances can effect the alkylation of molecules in the cell. It is common to them all that they can inhibit the growth of the cell. Among alkylating substances there are, in addition to nitrogen mustard, triethylene-melamine (TEM), which had already been developed during the war in Germany at the Farbwerke Hoechst. Clearly nobody at first saw in this compound an anti-cancer agent. TEM was, in fact, used in the textile industry to make materials crease-proof. The fact that it inhibits the growth of cells was only discovered in the fifties in the United States after it had been found that, in the reactions of nitrogen mustard with water, ionisation of the chloride occurred, followed by the formation of ethylene immonium ions.

Later there followed yet other ethylene imine derivatives, such as triethylene phosphoramide (TEPA) and triethylene thiophosphoramide (Thio-TEPA). All these substances have about the same range of usefulness as the nitrogen mustard preparations, but their side effects appear to be somewhat less marked.

Paul Ehrlich gives the first hint

Possibly the ethylene imines could have been introduced into cancer therapy half a century earlier if notice had been taken in good time of hints given by the German research worker and Nobel Laureate Paul Ehrlich. Ehrlich, known to posterity almost exclusively as the discoverer of "salvarsan" and as the founder of the chemotherapy of infectious diseases, had also worked intensively in his Frankfurt laboratory on cancer. Like many scientists of his time, he believed a speedy victory over cancer to be possible, although he expected the much-desired "magic bullet" to have less effect against cancer than against pathogenic microbes.

Ehrlich knew that the campaigns against bacteria and cancer are two basically different things. Cancer cells are not, as are bacteria, foreign bodies that penetrate into the organism; cancer cells are the degenerate sisters of normal cells, differing numerically but not qualitatively from healthy cells.

Ehrlich had found in 1898, even before his discovery of salvarsan, the unusual pharmacological properties of the ethylene imines. Among many hundreds of substances that Ehrlich investigated, the ethylene imines showed a noteworthy destructive effect on cells which divided rapidly. "Unfortunately" wrote Dr. Peter Alexander of the Chester Beatty Institute in *The Scientific American*, "this observation really became known to scientists only when Ehrlich's publications were reprinted in 1956. If it had not been overlooked in the rich store of Ehrlich's research results, we should not have had to await a World War in order to become aware of the possibilities of the alkylating agents."

Efficiency through chemical reorganisation

Meanwhile, among the numerous alkylating agents, two more have achieved priority in cancer therapy: namely Busulfan (Myleran) developed in the Chester Beatty Institute in London, and used against myeloid leukaemia, and cyclophosphamide (Endoxan), a further development of nitrogen mustard.

With cyclophosphamide a special substance was produced. It acts, not in the form first introduced into the body, but only after chemical reconstruction therein. In this way malignant cells can be affected more strongly than healthy ones and damage to the white blood cells can be largely avoided. The leucopenia – the radical fall in the number of white blood cells unavoidable with the first nitrogen-mustard compounds – is kept, with this compound, within narrow limits. In patients treated with cyclophosphamide there is only rarely a reduction of the number of leucocytes to less than 2,000 per ccm. of blood. A slight leucopenia is not at all undesirable. It is even regarded by many cancer specialists as a clear confirmation of effective treatment.

The best clinical results with cyclophosphamide are chiefly obtained in lymphosarcomata, reticuloses, and chronic leukaemia, and also in tumours of the digestive tract. Acute leukaemia is, in contrast to chronic leukaemia, only rarely affected by it.

Cyclophosphamide (Endoxan) stems from the laboratories of the German pharmaceutical firm of ASTA in Brackwede. Another preparation came from Bayer in Leverkusen. A new compound "E.39" was synthesized by the chemists W. S. Petersen and W. Gauss, and was tested thoroughly by the late Nobel Prize Laureate Gerhard Domagk for its effectiveness in the inhibition of cancer. Like mustard gas, TEM or Thio-TEPA, it is an alkylating agent.

In the Leverkusen laboratories two different substances were combined with one another – ethylene-imine derivatives and quinone. It was known that each of these individual compounds inhibited the course of cell division. Bayer "E.39" showed its value, not only against some tumours of animals but also against human tumours, especially if the preparations could be brought directly into contact with the malignant cells – for example, in haemoblastoses, tumours of the eyelid or malignant tumours of the skin.

At first, considerable quatities of solvents for this preparation were required: ethyl alcohol and physiological saline, so as not to damage the walls of the veins. A complex chemical reconstruction led ultimately to a watersoluble preparation of equal efficacy, Bayer "E.39 soluble".

Naturally the Bayer chemists were not satisfied with this preparation although it showed such great promise. Experiments were carried out with many reconstructed compounds, and these led to preparation "X", which was far superior in its ability to inhibit tumours. In order to attack tumours in animals effectively, a dose only one tenth of that of "Bayer E.39" was needed. In even a dilution of 1:1 thousand millions, preparation "X" interrupted the division of human tumours in cultures.

Under the name "Preparation 3231" it passed the clinical test so successfully that in the autumn of 1961 it was possible to include it in the Bayer list of drugs. Under the name "Trenimon" it is often used today. But trenimon, like other drugs, does not guarantee a curative effect.

Where is the point of attack?

Naturally the investigator of cancer has long been concerned with the question of how the alkylating substances check cell growth. It is known that their action is quite similar to that of radiation energy: that they can, like X-rays, cause mutations in the cancer cell, can intervene in the process of cell division and kill certain cells directly and make others malignant. For this reason they have been called radiomimetic substances, that is to say, substances with an action like that of radiation. However, it has not yet been possible to explain in detail how their biological intervention in the interior of the cell takes place, because they can react with almost all the important cell constituents.

Moreover, the process of alkylation can occur at different points in the cell molecule, and there is in this respect a whole series of reactions which are relatively harmless to the cell. But at which points of which molecules can alkylation lead to far-reaching injuries?

According to researches so far carried out, if alkylating agents can combine with the acid groups (COOH) of the cell molecules, which occur in all the proteins and nucleic acids, then they exhibit a radiomimetic action. Further, it has been shown that substances whose molecules contain two or more alkylating groups are much more active than those which have only one such group. They inhibit cell growth more strongly and cause greater damage to the chromosomes.

Presumably such injuries occur when an alkylating agent reacts simultaneously with two cell molecules and brings about a cross-linkage between them. Perhaps, if such a cross linkage should affect two halves of a chromosome before division, they would then be unable to separate cleanly and the daughter cells would bear a correspondingly altered and abnormal inheritance.

In "cross-links" of this kind, the point of attack of the alkylating substances would naturally be the DNA in the chromosomes. It has already been shown experimentally that the alkylating substances have the ability to cause such "cross-linking" of the DNA.

It has, however, not yet been proved that such a process actually occurs in the living cell. Whether it plays a part in the conversion of a normal cell into a malignant one, must remain a speculation. However alluring theories of this kind are, the fact remains that even today, 20 years after the discovery of the effects of alkylating compounds, no definite statement can be made about their mode of action.

Twenty years after the successful conversion of a chemical war gas into an anti-cancer drug, after the synthesis of hundreds of other alkylating substances, it still has regrettably to be conceded that none of these compounds has become an effective anti-cancer drug, as many investigators had hoped after the introduction of nitrogen mustard.

None of these substances is actually specific. The distinction that they make between healthy and malignant cells is only a hairsbreadth, and they attack equally all cells that divide rapidly. If one tried to use them at the full dose necessary to destroy the last remaining cancer cells in the body, they would prove fatal to the patient.

Thus it is that treatment always remains inadequate, that temporary remissions are achieved, but no actual cures.

On the other hand, even such partial successes are an enormous advance compared with the inadequate chemical "weapons" of the past. With the exception of arsenic, no previous chemical agent had proved much more effective than the primitive resources of African witch doctors!

Cell poisons against cancer of the skin

The so-called antimitotics have proved themselves to be the most effective. These are chemical substances which can preferentially inhibit mitosis – cell division.

Colchicine and its derivatives are the best-known of these substances. A poison of the meadow saffron, colchicine is one of those alkaloids which were first synthesized after the Second World War. But the effect of this poison on plant cells had already been observed before: the number of chromosomes doubled and the plants began to grow enormously. In animals, too, colchicine caused similar effects.

Thus the idea arose of testing this alkaloid on cancer cells. Unfortunately it proved to be extremely poisonous, so there seemed at first to be no question of its use in the general treatment of cancer. In the local treatment of tumours, however, colchicine can play a definite part, especially if it is applied directly to the tumour as an ointment. The diseases against which this "anti-mitotic" is most effective are lymphogranulomatosis, reticulosarcomas and cancers of the skin, but the promising results obtained with it in skin cancer – one foreign clinic reported 96 per cent success – must be contrasted with the mainly negative results obtained with internal tumours.

Causes and inhibitors of cancer

In the thirties, Karl Heinrich Bauer had indicated new lines of research into anti-cancer substances. Bauer started from the apparent paradox that radiation which caused cancer was also able to cure it, as the X-ray treatment of tumours had meanwhile proved.

This fact was not contradictory to the mutation theory. If one believed that radiation caused mutations in germ cells and cancer in body cells, it was logical to interpret the effects on cancer cells also as mutations.

Chemicals, too, which act as mutagens on germ cells and are carcinogenic to body cells must also produce fatal mutations in cancer cells. In order to demonstrate this in practice, Bauer treated moribund patients suffering from cancer with the strongest chemical carcinogen then available – 3, 4 benzpyrene.

Among 22 cases of skin cancer, which admittedly were very conveniently situated, Bauer was able, either by direct injection or by external application, to effect clinical cures in seven cases.

Bauer therefore showed "that under favourable conditions, spontaneous cancerous tissues react similarly to substances which have a carcinogenic effect on the body as they do to the "carcinogenic" effect of X-rays: not all tumours can be influenced, but those which cannot tolerate the mutagenic substance degenerate so much that clinical cure results."

Clearly such superficial cancers of the skin can be cured more simply and surely by surgery, so Bauer did not continue this research. For him, "the question was positively answered. Chemical substances can convert normal cells into cancer cells by somatic mutations and can kill cancer cells by additional mutations."

Alexander Haddow was later able to use hydrocarbons to inhibit the growth of tumours in animals, and Charles Huggins cured women with carcinoma of the mammary glands by means of methylcholanthrene.

Treatment with hormones

In this treatment Huggins made use of a double action mechanism. The women were not only treated with methylcholanthrene; at the same time the ovaries and adrenal cortex were removed so as to eliminate hormone stimulation in the mammary gland tissues.

Huggins had here followed a therapeutic method which he first successfully demonstrated in 1941. Carcinoma which is dependent on hormones can be treated by eliminating the corresponding hormone and artificially administering antagonistic ones.

Huggins started from the familiar idea that cancer of the

prostate is caused by excessive production of the male hormone. This apparently was the reason why men castrated in their youth, only rarely suffer from this disease. If such cancer is indeed due to an excess of male hormone, then a reverse effect must be produced by female hormone!

Huggins had his greatest success with a patient with advanced cancer of the prostate. He was able to show that his conjecture had hit the target. The patient, castrated and treated with female hormone, was completely cured. He died 15 years later of a quite different disease.

In breast cancer, too, the removal of the sex glands and treatment with male hormone has proved favourable. But this treatment is only resorted to when there are already extensive metastases in bone, for here an operation confined to the site of the tumour hardly helps at all. After operative endocrinic treatment, however, some of the secondary tumours do disappear.

Unfortunately in these hormone-dependent cancers complete and permanent cure, such as that obtained by Huggins with his first patient, cannot always be attained. After two or three years new formations of the cancer and a reactivation of the metastases may occur.

This may be due to the fact that the adrenal cortex, which also provides sex hormones, gradually compensates for the loss of the sex glands. These "neohormones" then give a growth stimulus to the secondary tumours.

When the "master gland" is eliminated

But in this instance, too, science can wage a defensive battle. The tumours can be again repressed by the removal of the adrenal cortex and by eliminating the hypophysis. This is usually done by "paralysing" the glands with radioactive gold. This operation has been undertaken during the last ten years in large clinics.

Usually it is applied to mammary carcinoma with numerous metastases, in which standard operations can no longer succeed. But once the hormonal driving force of the hypophysis is removed, not only do the secondary tumours in many cases degenerate, but also the severely affected bone system can sometimes regenerate itself. Altogether, Professor Bauer sees the hormone treatment of cancers as "the greatest advance in the treatment of cancer since the introduction of X-rays".

But no permanent cures can be obtained with this form of treatment, which is restricted to certain forms of cancer. "The dependence on hormones is sooner or later lost, so that a genuine cure by means of hormones alone, even with continuous treatment, is possible only in a few cases" writes Professor Hermann Druckrey. But Huggins has in any case proved "that the cancer can generally be successfully treated with chemical remedies. Thus the spell cast by the supposed impregnability of cancer is broken". Hundreds of promising new compounds have been synthesized and tested.

Oxygen for malignant cells

The effects of the alkylating agents were first discovered more or less accidentally. But behind other compounds there was, from the very beginning, a clear biochemical concept. Thus the observation of the German biochemist Otto Warburg that cancer cells do not breathe oxygen, but get their energy from fermentation, had offered a promising treatment of cancer.

Was there not here a tempting possibility of changing cancer cells back into healthy cells by feeding them oxygen? Patients could be put into rooms in which pure oxygen was concentrated at a pressure of one or two atmospheres. This treatment has, in fact, proved beneficial in many other diseases; however, no lasting effect has been shown on cancer. Research workers of the Vanderbilt and Johns Hopkins University in the U.S.A. developed a chemical which would interrupt the fermentation process in cancer cells without hindering the oxygen respiration by normal cells. This proved capable of blocking fermentation in human cancer cells and inhibiting cell division, but when used on man it proved highly toxic.

At the same time it emerged that Warburg's thesis had no general validity: many cancer cells definitely persist during oxygen respiration while many normal cells prefer fermentation.

The 82-year-old cancer investigator therefore aroused considerable astonishment when, in London in the summer of 1966, he gave a paper "On the ultimate and the remote causes of cancer" and strongly reproached his medical colleagues. "The ultimate cause of cancer is the replacement of oxygen respiration by fermentation in the body cells" Warburg proclaimed. "This offers a successful treatment of cancer which unfortunately is not used."

Warburg's plan for the prevention of cancer involved supplementing food with large quantities of the active groups of respiratory enzymes, so as to reduce risks of the formation of metastases after operation. "In this way it will never be possible to restore the de-differentiated cancer cells, because the probability of a re-differentiation during the brief span of human life is next to nil. But the respiration of growing metastases will be increased by inhibiting their fermentation, and their growth will be restricted to such an extent that they become harmless."

Warburg's critics point out that while fermentation can be demonstrated in many cancer cells, it has never been possible to prove that fermentation increases as the result of a respiratory injury. "The experiments carried out by Professor Warburg on the production of cancer cells through injury to the respiration of normal cells have not yet confirmed," says Professor Erich Hecker, Director of the Biochemical Institute of the German Cancer Centre in Heidelberg. "These experiments, moreover, have been carried out in tissue cultures, in conditions which are not comparable to those in man."

In the German Centre for Cancer Research, less work is therefore done on the respiratory processes of cancer cells than on the biochemical processes in the cell nucleus. "We think," says Professor Hecker, "that studies of the biochemical processes connected with the nucleic acids can contribute considerably to knowledge of the true causes of cancer."

The great differences in the nature of carcinogenic factors, in the eyes of Hecker, – and many other scientists – make it appear very doubtful whether the change from normal into cancer cells is due to a single primary cause. "It is more likely that different primary effects and their consequences lead to a single result – cancer."

Sulphonamides mark the beginning

The investigators had greater success with another biochemical concept, the starting point here being the sulphonamides. The first compounds of this kind were synthesized by the two Bayer chemists Fritz Mietzsch and Josef Klarer, and their antibacterial activity was revealed by Gerhard Domagk.

Some years later, after their first dramatic success against pneumonia and blood poisoning had become known, the British biochemist D. Woods was able to formulate a convincing hypothesis about the action of these substances. Woods proved that the "sulfas" stopped the growth of bacterial cells because they possessed a great similarity to para-amino-benzoic acid. This acid is needed by bacteria, but not by human cells.

It is a chemical pre-product of folic acid, which belongs to the Vitamin B complex and is necessary to human and animal cells alike. Bacteria synthesize folic acid by way of para-amino-benzoic acid, but the human body cannot do this. It must obtain supplies from the food consumed.

Bacterial cells cannot distinguish between sulphonamides and para-amino-benzoic acids. They willingly take up sulphonamides, which then block the enzyme systems of the cells like a badly-fitting key in a lock. Compounds like the sulphonamides are therefore called antimetabolites, because they bring disorder to the cell metabolism.

Would it not also be possible to employ these "saboteurs" successfully against cancer? This question increasingly interested biochemists. The more they discovered about the nucleic acids and their (relatively) simply-constructed constituents, the higher their hopes rose.

Just before a cell starts its division, a particularly active synthesis begins in its interior. It applies to the basic constituents of nucleic acid (purine and pyrimidine), for the DNA must reproduce itself extensively in order to provide the daughter cells with exact copies of itself. Would it not be possible to modify these compounds slightly – minimally enough to outwit the cancer cells, but sufficiently to cause disorder in the cell mechanism and inhibit division?

First of all it was necessary to clear up one thing: Do the cells use small chemical constituents for the construction of the nucleic acid bases, adenine, guanine, thymine and cytosine, or do they use, "prefabricated" larger compounds? At first, research workers believed that the cells build up these bases from their fundamental constituents. But investigations with radioactively marked atoms showed that this is not so. If cells are given adenine or guanine, these bases are taken up whole and are used in the synthesis of the complete DNA.

Thus the way was open for the first antimetabolites in the battle against cancer. In the Sloan-Kettering Institute the first compound of this kind, 2, 6 diaminopurine, was tested. This was a close chemical relative of the DNA-base adenine. From the first, research went extremely successfully. In test tubes containing normal and cancer cells, this pseudo-adenine quickly destroyed only the malignant cells. The others were not damaged. "This was the first direct proof that chemical antimetabolites could specifically destroy cancer cells. It was a thrilling discovery," says a report of the Institute.

First hopes were in vain

This chemically "falsified" adenine gave outstanding results not only in the test tube, but also in experiments on animals. But it failed in the fight against human cancer cells. A 17-year-old girl was cured of leukaemia for some years by this compound; she married and had a child – but then the disease returned and could no longer be arrested. In other sufferers from leukaemia it was possible to bring about a few very short-lived improvements. Some patients did not react to it at all.

Despite this, the first antimetabolite acted as a tremendous stimulus to cancer investigators. At least it was known that the chosen path was the right one. And soon the moment came for the first great success for this kind of chemotherapy. Dr. Sidney Farber, of the Children's Hospital in Boston, had spent many years on the study of the relationships between leukaemia and the influence of nutrition. He and his colleagues thought that certain dietary factors could increase resistance to cancer. Ultimately Farber treated some children suffering from acute leukaemia with folic acid. But the success of this vitamin treatment was very dubious. The general condition of some children improved, yet it had to be admitted that the doses of vitamin had stimulated the multiplication of malignant white blood cells still more.

However, this was an important signpost. Could not substances which took the place of folic acid in the chemistry of the cell act in the opposite manner, by slowing down cell multiplication or bringing it to a standstill?

Farber obtained, from the American drug firm of Lederle, some compounds of "falsified" folic acid which in fact caused a dramatic retrogression of tumours in hens. Following this, the first human patient was a child already suffering from very advanced leukaemia. The doctor prophesied a "life expectancy of two to three weeks". The antifolic acid brought about an appreciable improvement; it prolonged the life of this small patient by many months.

Reprieve, but no cure

In other children, too, who had already been given up by the doctors, this preparation brought unexpected improvements. Most children recovered in a few weeks, and were able to go back to school or to the playground. Was aminopterine – as the new preparation was called – the curative agent for leukaemia? After the treatment none of the children showed any symptoms of disease.

However, in every case, the leukaemia returned, often months or even years later.

Pure folic acid and its antagonist aminopterine are chemically very much alike. People who are not chemists will not at first note any difference at all in the structural formulae of the two. Only after a second look is an OH group detected in folic acid, which is replaced in aminopterine by an NH_3 group. A similar close relationship to their genuine antagonists is also shown by the other antimetabolites. Whilst aminopterine represents a chemical "counterfeit" of folic acid, an essential vitamin, mercaptopurine is a faked constituent of the DNA molecule.

As has been already stated, the DNA molecule consists of a framework of ribose and phosphoric acid. Four different bases function as rungs in this spirally-shaped molecule. Their infinitely varied successions represent the chemical code for heredity and cell-life.

A chemical "double" for adenine

In 1950 investigators already knew enough about the synthesis of nucleic acid for the chemotherapeutic point of attack to be transferred to the interior of the cell. Biochemists of the New York Sloan-Kettering Institute, together with their colleagues of the Wellcome Research Laboratories, synthesized a new compound, 6-mercaptopurine, which was copied from the nucleic acid base adenine and was chemically only slightly different from it.

Even in the first experiments on animals it was proved that this "double of adenine" suppressed the growth of a series of animal tumours. The first human patients were children with acute leukaemia. Among these the result was almost more dramatic. Patients who had not responded at all to other treatments, reacted extremely favourably to 6-mercaptopurine; in many of them the symptoms of the disease disappeared completely.

In the Sloan-Kettering Institute it was naturally desired to explore the mode of action of this new cancer remedy. Was there after all a general chemical difference between cancer cells and normal cells? Did mercaptopurine exploit such a difference?

Earl Balis, one of the scientists of the institute, had little concrete material to start from in his research. It was only known that 6-mercaptopurine must somehow hamper the formation of both adenine and guanine in the nucleic acid synthesis of new cells. Therefore the adenine antagonists had been actually "created". Definite proof of this was that the effect of 6-mercaptopurine could be nullified by large doses of natural purines.

Enzymes control DNA-metabolism

In his further studies Balis used bacterial cells. They are easily cultivated in a test tube and can be easily observed. Radioactive purines were an additional aid. Balis fed the bacterial cells with them. As the research workers in the Sloan-Kettering Institute had already supposed, it was then easy to show that the bacterial cells eagerly take up the purines and incorporate them into their nucleic acid bases, adenine and guanine.

Balis furthermore observed that adenine could be used by the cells to make guanine – the reverse process was also possible – according to the metabolic needs of the cells at the time.

The picture of undisturbed purine synthesis was radically altered when Balis, with his colleague Doris Hutchinson, selected another species of bacterium. This was a strain against which 6-mercaptopurine was ineffective. Balis found that this special strain could not use the purines fed to it in the test tube. Measurements of the radioactive material showed no noteworthy activity in the nucleic acids of the cells.

The conclusion from this was that 6-mercaptopurine in sensitive cells does not act itself as an antagonist. This is already done by a preliminary stage of nucleic acid (a ribonucleide) into which 6-mercaptopurine was incorporated. To put it more accurately, the enzyme which made a ribonucleide out of 6-mercaptopurine by combining with the glycophosphate, was the same as the one that initiated the production of adenine and guanine. Cells resistant to 6-mercaptopurine were in turn structures which had lost a certain enzymatic function.

There was a second result to this series of researches in the Sloan-Kettering Institute. Normal and sensitive cells which were treated with 6-mercaptopurine lost their ability to convert adenine into guanine.

At the time of this discovery in 1957 something was already known about the enzyme mechanism which initiated the formation of these two important constituents of nucleic acid. It had become clear that the ribonucleides, guanine and adenine, were initially produced by the same series of enzymes. Only at the tenth stage of the enzymatic action did the successive enzymatic pathways fork in two different directions. One led to adenine, the other to guanine.

The preliminary stage common to adenine and guanine is a compound called inosic acid. From this acid the way leads, through two further enzymatic stages, either to adenine or guanine. A cell that seeks to convert the adenine into guanine or the guanine into adenine therefore finds it easy. To do this, it needs only to retrace the existing enzymatic pathway to the inosic acid crossroad, and then to follow the corresponding road. But 6-mercaptopurine blocks this conversion of one base into the other.

Balis and his colleagues concluded from this that the disturbing influence of this compound must be directed towards the four further enzymatic stages. Further investigations then showed that 6-mercaptopurine puts itself in the place of inosic acid by a kind of exchange process and thus the course of the next two enzymatic stages is prevented: the synthesis of adenine and of guanine is stopped.

This was a fascinating glimpse into the complicated enzymatic events in the synthesis of nucleic acid. But another question was even more important: why does 6-mercaptopurine act more strongly on tumour cells than on normal cells?

Where does the difference in metabolism lie?

Balis again had to undertake extensive studies. By laborious experiments he compared the enzyme system of a mouse tumour that reacted to 6-mercaptopurine with that of normal liver tissue which did not. Radioactive inosic acid was introduced into extracts of the tumour and also of the liver. The result was that the enzymes of the liver were able to produce adenine – nucleotides twice as quickly, and guanine nucleotides four times as quickly, as the enzymes of the tumour.

The report of the Sloan-Kettering Institute on this says: "It was possible, at least in this case, to discover a noteworthy difference in the metabolic system of normal and cancer cells."

As further researches showed, the same difference exists between normal white blood cells and those of people suffering from different forms of leukaemia. Nowadays, therefore, 6-mercaptopurine is used especially in the fight against this form of cancer.

In the Sloan-Kettering Institute 6-mercaptopurine is regarded purely as the forerunner of an improved series of drugs, and other compounds are at present being investigated. They should interfere even more intensively with the synthesis of the purine constituents of nucleic acids.

A new antimetabolite

Mercaptopurine inhibits the interpolation of purines into the DNA chain. On the other hand, another substance acts especially against the pyrimidines. These are the smaller bases in the nucleic acid molecule: cytosine and thymine. In contrast to the DNA molecule in the nucleus of the cell, the ribonucleic acids present in the cell plasma for protein synthesis contain, instead of thymine, the pyrimidine derivative, uracil.

Pyrimidine sub-units of the DNA and RNA are formed in a very different way from purines. The formation of the basic structure of pyrimidine proceeds quite independently of the formation of the sugar constituent. Only when both parts of the molecule have been formed, does a special enzyme see to it that they are brought together. The last steps in this stage of the synthesis depend on which of the three pyrimidines – cytosine, thymine or uracil – is to be formed.

Microbiologists still do not know the final details of the incorporation of pyrimidine constituents into the nucleic acids, but it seems to be established that uracil is first united with the corresponding sugar and then with the phosphates. By an ensuing change – the DNA has, as has already been mentioned, one oxygen atom less than the RNA – the conversion of ribonucleotide into a deoxyribonulcleotide occurs. Finally uracil as a ribonucleotide is converted into thymine by the addition of a methyl group.

Among the various pyrimidine-antimetabolites, 5-fluor-uracil 5-FU) has so far proved most effective in cancer therapy. This is the base uracil, present in RNA instead of thymine, in which the methyl group (CH_3) is replaced by fluorine. Here also the chemists have undertaken only a slight change in the molecule, but this is sufficient to prevent the formation of thymine in the synthesis of DNA.

The young American biochemist Dr. Charles Heidelberger, of the University of Wisconsin, succeeded with the help of the Swiss drug firm Hoffmann – La Roche, in introducing 5-FU into the chemotherapy of cancer. Like all cancer drugs so far in use, 5-FU is still far from being an actual cure for cancer. Moreover, it is relatively toxic in high doses. However, there are in the U.S.A. a number of cancer patients who have, thanks to treatment with 5-FU, been kept alive for years. They are patients with breast cancer, cancer of the bowel, tumours of the digestive organs or of the liver.

Finally it was discovered that 5-FU exerts its most powerful effect, not in the form in which it is given to the patient, but only after combination with the sugar-phosphate groups. So Heidelberger took up his work anew.

Again in collaboration with the Hoffmann – La Roche chemists, especially with Robert Duschinsky, he devised a combination of 5-FU with the sugar constituents of DNA. This preparation is apparently somewhat less toxic, but also, unfortunately, no more effective that 5-FU.

At present Heidelberger is working on new pyrimidine antimetabolites. "These can only be," he says, "improvements of existing chemotherapy. Therefore I am allergic to the overstrained word, breakthrough, in cancer research. We have certainly made many advances. I am firmly convinced that we shall one day bring cancer under control. But it is a dangerous nonsense to suggest to the general public that a cure awaits us round the next corner."

Why do cells become resistant?

Cancer investigators today are not only concerned with the development of new preparations. They are just as busy with the problem of resistance. This phenomenon had been already encountered in bacteria which become resistant to sulphonamides and to certain antibiotics.

There is also a resistance to chemotherapeutic substances among cancer cells. After a promising start, many preparations suddenly cease to prevent the development of tumours. "The body has become resistant," many laymen say of this process.

Actually this is true neither of the sulphonamides and antibiotics, nor of the chemical agents against cancer. Treatment with antibiotics does not make the organism resistant. When the sensitive bacteria are killed, only the non-susceptible ones remain. Their multiplication is then unchecked. Ultimately they inundate the whole organism if another antibiotic is not administered in time.

It is similiar with cancer cells. As the American cancer investigator V. R. Potter, Professor of Oncology in the McArdle Memorial Institute writes: "it is known that most tumours consist of a mixture of cells of different kinds. Some of them are sensitive, and others resistant, to a certain drug, so that only the sensitive strains disappear under treatment." The surviving cancer cells multiply further, until ultimately the whole tumour consists only of their daughter cells. A resistant tumour has been formed.

Because the cells in an individual tumour can thus be quite different, daughter tumours, unlike their progenitor, often do not respond to certain drugs. "Metastases were formerly considered to be merely a displacement and multiplication of cells of a primary tumour," writes Professor Hans Lettré. "But the latest observations show that there can also be a selection of cell-lines with altered characteristics."

But why are many cells resistant to certain drugs from the very start? This is explained at present by the loss of certain enzymes which are necessary for the effective conversion of the drug in the interior of the cell. The loss of these enzymes might have occurred during the development of a malignant cell, but can also be the result of a mutation, through which from time to time new kinds of cells are formed.

Other causes are also possible. Malignant cells are often quite flexible. Whilst they are at first sensitive to a cancer drug, they learn, in course of time, to adjust their metabolic processes. In this way, they procure for themselves the raw materials necessary for their synthesis.

Another means of survival is a kind of stockpiling of reserves. The cancer cells store up the materials required for their synthesis, and in spite of the blockade by the drug, they can continue to satisfy their metabolic requirements.

Interplay of drugs

Cells resistant to a particular compound often react all the more sensitively to a different one. Thus cancer therapeutists have devised a well-thought-out interplay of different drugs. Combinations of chemotherapeutics are made to act as effectively as possible on cancer cells with one onslaught, and thereby to prevent the selection and formation of less sensitive cells. Nowadays, for example, four or five different preparations are often used simultaneously against leukaemia: possibly mercaptopurine, folic acid antagonists, corticosteroids and the alkaloid vincristin.

The history of vincristin began, as has so often happened in pharmaceutical research, in a field of work that had nothing to do with cancer. The American Dr. James Harry Cutts and his colleagues in the University of Western Ontario, had originally been concerned with an extract of a tropical plant, to which medicine-men in South Africa and the Philippines had ascribed the ability to reduce blood sugar.

When the American research team tested this extract in experiments on animals, they found that, in rats and mice, the number of white blood cells was for some days greatly reduced. This effect, however, was transitory, and quite soon the white blood cells became even more numerous. Moreover, the extract inhibited leukaemia transmitted to animals, as well as solid tumours transplanted into them, and slowed down the growth of some spontaneous tumours.

On the basis of this research, two preparations were then developed – vincristin and vinblastin. In spite of their marked side effects, they are nowadays used for some kinds of human cancer, including choriocarcinoma, cancers of the lungs and stomach, and lymphomas, as well as for some forms of leukaemia. They have a strong effect, but this often lasts only a short time.

Antibiotics against cancer cells

Some antibiotics have also secured for themselves an important place in the treatment of cancer. These are metabolic products of mould fungi (Hyphomycetes) or Actinomyces, which act on bacteria as metabolic poisons and have become some of the most active weapons against infectious diseases. It has later been discovered that some of them can inhibit the growth of certain tumours; this is especially true of Actinomycin, the active substance of strains of Actinomyces and Streptomycetes.

A research team of the Organic Chemistry Institute of the University of Göttingen, under its Director Professor Hans Brockmann, carried out thorough researches in this field. This team discovered Actinomycin C, which, because it was extremely toxic in animal experiments was at first thought inadmissible in human medicine.

Brockmann and his colleagues succeeded in working out the structure of Actinomycin C and ultimately in synthesizing it. This showed that it was a completely new antibiotic, consisting of a peptide constituent and a pigment, the so-called chromophor. The chromophor constituent is always the same in the various actinomycins, which differ only in their different peptide constituents.

The antibiotic effect of the actinomycins depends on their ability to combine with the DNA of the cells affected. How this occurs is still unknown, but it is certain that the actinomycins occupy parts of the DNA matrices. The result of this is that the DNA loses the ability to form some kinds of RNA, especially the messenger-RNA that is so important in the events occurring in the cell.

This mode of attack is certainly responsible for the effect of Actinomycin C on tumour cells. It has, for example, been shown to damage various tumours inoculated into animals, and it acts especially on lymphogranulomatosis, or "Hodgkin's Disease". Intravenous doses of Actinomycin C can occasionally produce improvements in this disease.

Success with the Wilms – tumour

The Memorial Hospital of the Sloan-Kettering Institute in New York has achieved considerable success in the treatment of so-called Wilms-tumours in children by means of Actinomycin D. These are rapidly-growing tumours of the kidney which mainly form metastases in the lobes of the lungs. Within about eleven months from the first symptoms they lead to death, whatever is done in the way of radiotherapy, surgery or chemotherapy.

Many parents and children were able to gather fresh hope when, about ten years ago, the first series of researches with actinomycin was started. Since then a total of 72 children have been treated in the Memorial Hospital with the new drug, and 13 of them are still alive today. These 13 children all had lung-metastases, which completely disappeared in nine of the young patients. Of these nine, after periods of four to to eight years, six are still quite free from all signs of tumour. In the other three, in whom the tumours have completely undergone involution, only one to 1½ years has passed since the cure.

Another antibiotic, Mitomycin C, is also used in cancer therapy, particularly in Japan. Its mode of action is, however, still unknown and no definite opinion can yet be expressed about its chances of success.

New possibilities also seem to be revealed by combined treatment with X-rays and doses of antibiotics. The first successes were reported to a medical congress in Toronto by radiologist Marvin Lougheed and surgeon Dr. John Palmer of the Montreal General Hospital in Canada. Lougheed and Palmer were dealing in their work with sarcomas of the bones in limbs. X-ray treatment cannot in general achieve much with such tumours. Effective treatment requires such high doses of radiation that the functional efficiency of the limb itself is lost, so that often only amputation can bring deliverance.

But the two Canadian doctors now found that a combination of radiation and treatment with the antibiotic Actinomycin D offered chances of avoiding a radical operation. Like Actinomycin C, Actinomycin D probably combines with the DNA of the cell nucleus to form an as yet unknown substance which makes the cells more sensitive to radiation. In particular, it "renews" the effect of radiation after this has died away. This makes it possible to treat patients with much smaller doses of radiation than would otherwise be necessary.

By Palmer and Lougheed's method, the patient is first irradiated repeatedly for 3½ weeks from a cobalt source, in which the total amount of radiation is 4,500 rad. After this the arteries which supply the tumour are suffused for half an hour with

Actinomycin D. Later, at intervals of 1 week each two further irradiations with a total dose of 2,500 rad are given.

According to the Montreal report, this method was used in 10 patients. One of them was beyond help. Two of them still had to suffer an amputation. But seven of them were still alive after periods of 3 months to 3½ years, and free from metastases.

Help from heart-lung machines

Treatment of cancer with drugs – often combined with surgery and X-ray treatment – has, without doubt, improved continuously. New methods of application also play their part. As with X-ray treatment, the problem has been to restrict the action of the drug as much as possible to the tumour. Other tissues, especially the blood-building bone marrow, must be fully protected. Cytostatics exert their inhibitory and destructive effect on normal and malignant cells alike; the method of treatment must therefore be arranged so as to apply these substances directly to the tumour.

In doing this the surgeon is an indispensable help to the chemotherapist. Among procedures which have developed from this co-operation is the technique of infusion. The cytostatic is led through a catheter directly into the arteries which supply the tumour. It then develops its strongest effect on the cancer tissue. Obviously this method cannot wholly prevent it from reaching the surrounding tissues and ultimately the general circulation.

Still better control can be attained by the complex technique of perfusion, in which that part of the body in which the tumour lies is temporarily cut off from the general circulation. It is supplied with an artificial circulation by means of a heart-lung machine. The cytostatic is then introduced into this separate system. But the treatment then lasts for some 1½ hours; the method can therefore only be used in certain cases, such as in tumours of the extremities, since it is generally too difficult in the pelvic region, the breast, the head and neck.

New techniques, with the aid of which the blood platelets can be renewed in order to avoid haemorrhages and the exchange of white blood cells, are also some of the refined methods of treatment with which an extension of life expectancy can be attained, especially in leukaemia.

Professor Georges Mathé, Director of the Institut de Cancérologie et Immunogénétique in Villejuif, near Paris, has taken an important step, beyond even these methods of treatment. After attempts had been made since 1958 in France and America to treat leukaemia by the transfusion of bone marrow, Mathé and his colleagues succeeded, in the spring of 1963, in so curing a leukaemia patient. The patient was a doctor, aged 27, who had suffered since the summer of 1961 from severe leukaemia.

The bone marrow transfusion, during which a total quantity of 2,000 cc of bone marrow was injected into the veins, lasted about two hours. Even after two days, it could be seen that restoration of the bone marrow had begun. The transfused marrow came from the young doctor's parents, from his sister and his three brothers.

Although the bone marrow used came from near relatives, the doctor was twice irradiated, some days before the transfusion, with Cobalt 60 in order to suppress his immune reaction against the foreign bone marrow. Because there is, in this method, a risk of very severe infections, the patient was completely isolated and kept under aseptic conditions until he was discharged. When, in the summer of 1963, he left the hospital, his blood was completely free from leukaemia cells.

By January, 1966, Professor Mathé had succeeded in the same way with another case. This time it was a girl 17 years old. "She was suffering from leukaemia in its last stage," reported Professor Mathé. "Also her condition was extremely critical after the transfusion. Just look at these temperature charts. We had to contend for weeks with temperatures of 104 degrees to 106 degrees F. But today the patient is in splendid condition."

Mathé took us to the sickroom. The corridor was continually irradiated with ultraviolet light to kill infective organisms. The girl lay behind a thick glass partition. She sat up in bed and laughed when Mathé spoke to her over the room telephone. Jokingly she removed the white bonnet from her head to show how some of her hair had fallen out as a result of the preceding irradiation. This girl had also received bone marrow from near relatives, but from three other donors as well. Perhaps it was these that caused the severe reaction to the transfusion.

Professor Mathé has still not progressed far enough to be able to say what prospects there are for this treatment for leukaemia. "Our experience is still much too limited. We feel almost as if we're playing the part of space explorers who shoot a satellite into the cosmos and then must await developments."

Nevertheless, these bone marrow transfusions are of great scientific interest. Perhaps they will prove to be decisive means for the investigation of relationships between viruses and human leukaemia.

"At present there is no proof that human leukaemia is caused by viruses, as has been certainly proved in animals. We cannot infect man with suspect viruses and then wait to see whether leukaemia develops or not."

But in Mathé's institute the rôle of research subjects will be taken in future by rhesus monkeys. Some time ago Mathé succeeded in transfusing bone marrow between animals of the same genus, i.e. from mice to other mice. Transfusion of rat bone marrow to mice also succeeded. "We have thus," said Mathé, "made rats produce the bone marrow of mice."

The next great step will be transfusion of human bone marrow to monkeys. If this succeeds, the bone marrow in these monkeys should produce human blood cells. Utimately the animals will be inoculated with leukaemia viruses. If these human blood cells in the monkeys then develop leukaemia, conclusive proof may exist that some forms of human leukaemia, at least, are caused by viruses.

American research workers also expect human leukaemia to provide the means for a great breakthrough in the campaign against cancer. In the United States, therefore, research efforts are increasingly directed towards this form of cancer. The American Cancer Society alone has devoted in recent years at least 12 million dollars to a special leukaemia research programme. Several hundred million dollars have hitherto been invested in the screening of compounds that inhibit cell growth.

In the past 10 years, no fewer than 221,000 chemical and vegetable substances from all parts of the world have been tested for their effect against cancer. Of this impressive number, 285 compounds passed initial tests and qualified for the first clinical trials. Thousands of patients voluntarily made themselves available for this purpose.

Among these substances, there was in fact no effective anti-cancer preparation. But who can say whether such a substance will not one day be found? Dr. Kenneth M. Endicott, who, as Chief of the National Cancer Institute, directs American strategy in the campaign against cancer, takes as his battle-cry: "The search must go on."

Chapter 7

SEEKERS AFTER NEW WAYS

In 1866 in Berlin, Doctor Busch made an interesting discovery. It seemed to indicate a completely new course for the campaign against cancer. Busch had to treat a patient who had, to all appearances, only a short time to live. His case history was one of numerous sarcomas. All other findings showed that the malignant growths were progressing rapidly. Then the man also developed traumatic erysipelas, owing to a streptoccocal infection of the skin. It was not possible at that time to treat either the cancer or the infection with any medicaments then known. Busch could only wait till fate irrevocably put an end to the double disease.

However, it turned out quite differently. The development of the tumour, which should, according to all observations have continued unchecked, slowed down and suddenly came to an end. The malignant tumours underwent involution and fused together.

Naturally the question arose as to whether there could be a relationship between this spontaneous recovery and the simultaneous appearance of the erysipelas. Was it possible that the streptococci which caused the erysipelas, had attacked and destroyed the tumour cells?

The idea was tempting enough to prompt the most meticulous investigations into cancer and traumatic erysipelas. By laborious work over a decade the German cancer investigator Erich Huth worked to collect the histories of cases that had suffered simultaneously from these two diseases. He found 46 cases in which sarcoma or carcinoma had developed together with traumatic erysipelas. In seven of these sarcomas and six of the carcinomas there had been permanent recoveries – which only normally occur in one in a hundred thousand cases.

Now the scientists went a step further. They infected incurable cases of cancer with streptoccocci. This clearly showed that this new treatment, at first sight so hopeful was subject to an inadmissible risk: there was as yet no effective agent against these bacteria. The era of the sulphonamides and antibiotics had not yet dawned, and it was impossible to control the artificially induced bacterial infection. The patients died of it even before the cancer could complete its destructive work. Nor did extracts of streptococci provide the answer, for the state of bacteriology and biochemistry at that time did not permit the making of standardised and stable preparations.

Therefore, in the course of further experiments, efforts were made to attack the cancer cells by other less dangerous micro-organisms. Using intestinal bacteria, parasites and organisms belonging to the intermediate stages between bacteria and viruses – nowadays classified as mycoplasmas – attempts were made to obtain less dangerous extracts.

Again and again it was possible to record an inhibitory effect on tumour cells, and in experiments on animals, even actual recoveries. The results, however, were neither numerous nor conclusive enough to justify investigating the use of micro-organisms on a broader basis.

Treatment with viruses

The more scientists worked on viruses, the nearer also came the idea of using these particles, which only multiply in living cells, against cancer. Was there a possibility of mobilising one enemy of mankind against another? Recently American doctors have achieved important improvements by injecting leukaemia patients with suspensions of viruses. Even after a few days there were astonishing results: the uncontrolled production of white blood cells declined, the severe pains in the liver disappeared. The haemorrhages in the mucosae of the nose and mouth ceased and the enlargements of the liver, spleen and lymph glands decreased.

However – as unfortunately always happens with cancer – these effects only lasted for a short time. The disease was restrained, but not cured. In the duel between virus and cancer, the malignant cells remained the victors.

For all that, at least a reprieve was achieved. In what way was this possible? If leukaemia is regarded as a virus infection, the process can be interpreted, under certain conditions, as a displacement effect. The "old" leukaemia viruses, so to speak, uphold their domestic authority in the cells they affect. They defend themselves against the new invaders. A war develops between the two kinds of virus. If it ends victoriously for the invaders, which are not causes of cancer, the organism can then count on a certain respite in the course of the disease.

Here also, as in all spheres of previous cancer research, the calculations of the research workers proved to be in the highest degree imperfect. It gradually became clear that there was only the briefest possible contact between the carcinogenic viruses and the cells. As Dr. Michael Stoker, of the distinguished Virus Institute of the University of Glasgow wrote: "During this contact the virus can, under certain conditions, alter the hereditary structure of the cell, without its further presence being necessary."

In other words: the virus channels its DNA into the cell and, "grafts" an additional DNA on to the cell nucleus. The virus DNA is thus an irregular constituent of the hereditary substance of the affected cells, which then either die or multiply further with the foreign inheritance. The virus itself is no longer present, but its DNA has become a constituent of the malignant cells. Naturally in such cases the chances of combating cancer by means of artificial infections with harmless viruses are not very high.

Now, however, another possibility is conceivable. There are viruses which by preference multiply in tumours. What happens if viruses of this kind – such, perhaps, as the "Egypt virus 101" – are injected into tumours, which are then used as breeding places for enormous quantities of virus material? Workers in the New York Sloan-Kettering Institute spent much time on research of this kind without any practical result. "We have not," says Dr. David Karnofski of the New York Institute, "completely abandoned our work in this sphere, but at present we do not expect very much from it."

Tumours disintegrated from within

On the other hand, some years ago, bacilli played an interesting part in the search for biological controls of cancer. This involved spores of bacteria which only develop in an anaerobic environment, such as, for example, in a cancer cell which is poor in oxygen.

Every cell requires energy for its innumerable biochemical processes. In normal cells this happens by respiration – they burn carbohydrates in an oxygen environment (i.e. aerobic conditions) into carbon dioxide and water. Many cancer cells on the other hand, use another method of getting energy. Dispensing with oxygen (under anaerobic conditions) they break down the glucose nutrient in the blood into lactic acid. In this process of fermentation every kind of respiration is, so to speak, "forbidden". It always effects only an incomplete breakdown of the carbohydrate into lactic acid. It is this abnormal metabolism which – it is thought – gives the cancer cells their extraordinary energy, and promotes their virulence .

This was already known in 1923, thanks to Otto Warburg, who was awarded the Nobel Prize for his work on respiratory enzymes. According to Warburg's incessantly propagated theory which for the first time proclaimed a fundamental biochemical difference between healthy and malignant cells, the normal cell is deprived by certain chemicals or by irradiation of the ability to gain energy from respiration. In the battle for survival, cells thus damaged ultimately switch over to fermentation. They retain this habit, even when oxygen is available and the poisonous substances no longer act on them.

If Warburg's theory is correct, the change from health to malignancy would be plausible, as also would be the long latent period before cancer tumours show themselves in man. In fact many experiments have succeeded in causing cells in cultures, to change their metabolism to fermentation by depriving them of oxygen and in this way to convert them into cancer cells.

Unfortunately this impressive theory had in subsequent decades to undergo some important modifications.

By no means all cells which become malignant change from breathing oxygen to anaerobic fermentation. But even in cells which undergo this metamorphosis, scientists are by no means agreed as to the result or the cause. Many of them think that the change to fermentation is not the long-sought primary process in the origin of cancer, but is only a frequent result of it.

Spores prefer less oxygen

It remains clearly undisputed that many tumour cells ferment. A phenomenon also long known to science was that the spores of certain groups of bacteria grow into their vegetative form, the rods, only in an environment poor in oxygen. Among these are the widely ramified families of bacilli, the Clostridia. These spore-forming micro-organisms are not only common in soil, but also in the digestive tract of man and animals. Some of them are harmless parasites, many are useful in industry, but among them are also numerous species of pathogenic Clostridia, such as *Clostridium tetani*, the cause of traumatic tetanus. Common to them all is the fact that they are anaerobic.

Quite independently of Warburg's observation of anaerobic glycolysis, the hygienist, Josef R. Möse, arrived at a new biological point of departure in the treatment of cancer. Professor Möse originally wished simply to demonstrate to his students that tetanus spores were harmless to mice. Because no healthy mice were available to him, he used mice with tumours. Unexpectedly the mice died of traumatic tetanus. But healthy mice did not react at all to intravenous injections of tetanus spores. For the tetanus spores did not find anywhere in the healthy cells the anaerobic conditions under which to develop. In the cells of animals with tumours, on the other hand, anaerobic fermentation provided the spores with ideal conditions for growth. They were able to develop into bacteria and their toxins caused tetanus in the animals.

Now, however, as has already been mentioned, there are various species of Clostridia that are harmless to man and animals alike. Möse eventually encountered *Clostridium butyricum*, which is related to the tetanus bacilli but is, however, quite harmless to man and animals.

Suspensions of the spores of this bacillus were injected into normal animals and those suffering from cancer. The healthy animals showed no special reactions. But in those with tumours, a noteworthy phenomenon was recorded. Originally the tumours were hard and compact. Suddenly they became soft and watery (serous). Ultimately the fluid began to break through to the outside with the dead cells: the tumour in a few days had completely disintegrated.

Small tumours are unresponsive

In a tumour disintegration of this kind large crater-like tissue defects arise. As happens with burns, the body is flooded and poisoned by decomposition products. This flooding cannot sucessfully be prevented either by antihistamine preparations or by corticosteroids or vitamins. The animals therefore die of them. But perhaps latent infections, activated by the dissolution of the tumour, also play a part.

Obviously these breakdown products are a greater danger to small experimental animals than to man, because the relationship between the size of the animal and the size of the tumour is extremely unfavourable. In animals the tumour may amount to about a fifth of the volume of the body. In man the ratio is 1.70. On the other hand the oncolysis is possible only in larger tumours. Most small tumours do not react. They are too well supplied with Clostridia find it hard to develop. An important requirement for blood, and oxygen respiration in the cells is still largely intact; in such an environment the spores cannot settle down and germinate.

These conditions occur also in many tumours of external regions, where cells at the perimeter are still well supplied with blood and are capable of intensive growth; in these, too, the Clostridia find it hard to develop. An important requirement for development, incidentally, seems to be that sufficient disintegrated cancer tissue should be already present as a "nutrient medium" for the spores.

Researches on animals had already shown that different kinds of animal tumour react differently to Clostridia. Golden hamsters, for example, are highly sensitive, and tumours in these can be completely disintegrated by even small doses of spores. Rats, on the other hand, are almost completely resistant; it has been shown that rat-serum has a destructive effect on Clostridia.

First researches on man

For the first time people suffering from cancer have been treated with Clostridia. Naturally these have only been patients regarded as absolutely incurable. No one could say in advance whether human tumours could also be disintegrated, or whether man could tolerate the injection of spores.

Professor Möse discovered the answer in work on 36 cancer patients. It was that the spores dissolve tumours not only in animals but also in man. The individual patients were given 3.5–28 milliard spores, and in none of the cases were there noteworthy side effects.

Other doctors have since used Clostridia in the campaign against cancer, and have treated patients suffering from brain tumours, gynaecological tumours and certain sarcomas. They, too have been able to record the dissolution of tumours in a series of patients. But other malignant tumours hardly reacted. This resistance had already been frequently observed in experiments in animals, probably because the Warburg thesis is incomplete. Cancer cells which have not switched to fermentation do not offer suitable environment for spore growth. Thus lyses are not possible. But, even where tumour cells had actually been disintegrated, it was occasionally observed that the rods of the bacilli reverted to the inactive spore form, at which point the process of disintegration came to a halt. This is presumably connected with the fact that, in the course of the tumour breakdown, certain substances (porphyrines) are liberated which promote the reversion of the rod to the inactive spore form. This unwelcome intervention of the porphyrines can be prevented to a large extent by an elegant biological trick. Porphyrine readily combines with heavy metals. Thus it can be made inactive by the administration of certain heavy metal compounds such as, for example, iron-dextran complex.

Another observation was still more vital. Even when by far the greater part of a tumour had disintegrated, small residues of malignant cells remained. They formed the starting point for a new growth.

Brain tumours react sensitively

It is difficult to foretell what kinds of tumours will respond to the spores, for unfortunately tumour material taken by biopsy cannot be tested beforehand in a test tube. However, it seems that brain tumours react most sensitively to the Clostridia, which are injected directly into them via the nearest arteries. Whether lysis then occurs depends essentially on how well the tumour area is supplied with blood vessels.

The place of oncolysis in the future campaign against cancer can still not be forecast. For the time being it can only be said that it represents an attempt to attack the cancer problem from its outskirts, which is as fascinating as it is unorthodox.

Although many of the results obtained hitherto are so encouraging, the statement made by Dr. Dietmar Gericke director of the Hoechst cancer laboratory in his summary of research to the end of 1965, cannot be ignored: "So far it has not been possible to cure any case; intact tumour tissue has always been found in the transition zone to normal tissue."

Perhaps these dangerous remains of the tumours can be "smoked out" by combined treatment with chemotherapeutic substances. In the United States, in the laboratories of Merck, Sharp and Dohme, early experiments have been done on this in close collaboration with Professor Möse and Farbwerke Hoechst. Among the many substances tested, 5-fluor-uracil proved to be the most effective. Work has also been done on a combination of oncolysis and X-ray treatment.

At the same time the search for other strains of Clostridia naturally continues. Perhaps there are Clostridia which carry out the destruction of tumours more thoroughly still, or perhaps existing strains can be made more aggressive by various biological procedures.

How does the biological mechanism which causes tumour disintegration actually work? In spite of intensive research, this is not yet known in detail. At first it was thought that the Clostridia produced a kind of antibiotic, but this has not been confirmed.

At present, two other hypotheses exist. In oncolysis the tumour cells and the Clostridia must compete for the cell nutrients. In this struggle the Clostridia hold the field at the expense of the cancer cells. But it could also be possible that one of the enzymes produced by the Clostridia has cell-destroying properties – though it is still certain that the spores can do nothing against healthy cells. Only the tumour tissue, with its anaerobic conditions, offers them a point of attack, and spores which do not reach the source of nutrition die off. They are destroyed without any injurious effect; the richness of the healthy cells in oxygen simply offers them no chance of life.

"The decisive feature of this method seems to us to be," said Dr. Gericke, "that we can, by oncolysis, effect a direct attack on the tumour in which no normal tissue will be destroyed. It is, however, clear that our results so far are only a beginning, and that much must still be done before a clinical treatment can be devised. Even then, in operable tumours, the surgeon's knife will take precedence over oncolysis."

Cure by hot baths

Researches in 1965 tended towards the biological rather than the physical, and also provided extensive headlines for the press. They concerned a relatively new means of treating cancer by hyperthermia, or overheating. When Manfred von Ardenne reported these researches at the end of the 1965, on the celebration of the 75th birthday of Professor Bauer in Heidelberg University, he shocked his illustrious audience into scarcely concealed scepticism.

Cancer cells are much more sensitive to heat than healthy cells. In tissue cultures, the German cancer investigator H. Vollmar was able, as early as 1941, to show that temperatures of 104 degrees to 108 degrees F. cause marked injury to cancer tissue but do not affect healthy tissues. Many of the rare spontaneous cures of tumours point in the same direction. About 150 cases are known in which, after an acute disease accompanied by very high fever, a cancerous tumour spontaneously underwent involution.

The sensitivity of cancer cells to heat was therapeutically investigated as long ago as 1910. At that time, carcinomas of the skin, which are readily accessible, were treated with hot water.

The Erlangen surgeon O. Goetze went a step further. In cases of carcinoma of the penis and melanosarcomas of the limbs, he ligatured the affected member and thus produced a hyperthermia. Then he anaethetised the patient and exposed the affected part to great overheating. This was repeated several times. In this way Goetze actually succeeded in curing the tumours completely, and in maintaining the cure for years.

However, the use of this method is very limited. It is applicable only to tumours in the limbs, which are very rare. But it is useless if metastases have already been formed.

In order to reach such secondary tumours by treatment with hyperthermia, a more thorough procedure is necessary, and the patient's whole body must be greatly overheated. But in this there are difficulties which many decades of technical work have not overcome. It was especially necessary to avoid damage to the brain cells which are very sensitive to high temperatures.

The physicist Manfred von Ardenne therefore constructed a complicated apparatus, which made overheating to 112 degrees F. possible. The anaesthetised patient was put into a bath divided into two compartments. His body from feet to neck lay in a "hot" compartment, into which water could be led at will for heating or cooling. The upper part of the neck and the head, on the other hand, lay in a "cold' compartment, in order to prevent too great a strain on the brain.

It is reported that von Ardenne has already treated 48 patients in this apparatus at the Dresden University Surgical Clinic. They were overheated repeatedly for periods of half to threequarters of an hour, some to 108 degrees F. and, in a few cases, even to 110 degrees F. In this way tumours the size of a child's head were reduced to the size of a hen's egg in six weeks. One cannot therefore speak of complete cures, only of improvements, but patients can be given some additional years of life until perhaps having to undergo another course of similar treatment.

Probably this treatment can only be applied at present to relatively young people with a good constitution, for the overheating is a very great strain on the circulation. Besides, in some tumours other complications may arise. Thus, in the Dresden Institute, two deaths were recorded of patients with sarcomas. Sarcoma, as it happens, seems to disintegrate especially rapidly under overheating. The result of this is that the body is suddenly flooded with toxic products which it can no longer tolerate.

Nevertheless, Manfred von Ardenne will not let hyperthermia go at that. His basic idea is treatment by successive stages, in which the overheating could be combined with chemotherapeutic treatment.

Ardenne's work here has not yet progressed beyond the stage of experiments on animals. At first he worked with tissue cultures of ascites-cancer cells from mice. It was known that a chemical compound, DL-glycerine aldehyde selectively kills such cells. However the richer the affected tumour was in cells, the more quickly the effect of glycerine aldehyde waned. Ardenne found that the external cells of the tumour "used up" the drug too vigorously, so that the internal cells were no longer reached.

But when Ardenne first heated his tissue cultures, he was able to discover that the consumption of the drug declined significantly. If the heat was raised for half an hour to 108 degrees

F. the consumption of the drug was reduced to a sixth, and with a rise to 112 degrees F. even to a 26th.

According to Ardenne, experiments on animals later showed that the effect of the drug is increased about ten times after hyperthermia.

On this Ardenne based his hope of developing a treatment of cancer by several stages. According to his theory, about 95 per cent of the cancer cells could be killed by hyperthermia. Thereafter, chemotherapeutic treatment must be used. With its help an additional 4 per cent of the malignant cells could, perhaps, be successfully destroyed.

This would not, however, suffice for a definite cure, for which it would be necessary to destroy the cancer cells in the ratio of 100,000 : 1. But a quota of 100 : 1, Ardenne thought "corresponds in tumours of medium malignity to a lengthening of life of up to two years". After this period the tumour must be again treated by the same method. Ardenne considered that the time could definitely come when patients "live with cancer", just as nowadays they do with diabetes.

Only in the stage of research

At present, however, such thoughts are dreams of the future. Ardenne himself emphasized that "it must be strongly emphasized that our investigations in Dresden are still at the exploration stage. A large programme of work will probably keep us busy for years before the proposed treatment of cancer can be used in medical practice."

There is still no indication, even in outline, of which tumours will respond to treatment of this kind and which will not. In addition, the patient under hyperthermia must also have a completely healthy and resistant circulation.

Among cancer investigators in the Federal Republic of Germany many disparaging criticisms have been expressed. It has also been pointed out that similar methods of heating were used on inoperable tumours many years ago by Professor Heinrich Lampert in the Weserberg Clinic in Höxter. Ardenne's work is therefore by no means new.

The three chief weapons against cancer – surgery, chemotherapy and radiology – have not at present been significantly extended by hyperthermia. On the other hand, this is not so of the immunological methods of treating cancer which nowadays occupy much space in cancer research and have already yielded many hopeful results. The American National Cancer Institute, the Sloan-Kettering Institute in New York, and the laboratories of the French Institute of Scientific Research on cancer are especially occupied with these problems.

The research report of the Sloan-Kettering Institute for November 1965 said: "there is today no reliable indication that certain forms of human cancer can be overcome by means of antibodies". However, it seems increasingly likely that a "fourth" weapon against cancer is already in sight.

Chapter 8

WHEN THE IMMUNOLOGICAL SYSTEM FAILS

"Volunteers required for cancer experiments," said the headline in the *Ohio Penitentiary News*. These were the first experiments to see whether cancer can be transmitted from one human being to another. In this way scientists hoped to discover how it is that cancer occurs in some people and not in others. Why it is the fate of only one out of six persons, and why 85 per cent of the population are exempt from the scourge of our century. Whether one man can resist cancer while others cannot, and whether there is such a thing as immunity to cancer.

From the nineteenth century German doctor A. von Hanau, who founded experimental cancer research with his experiments on rats, all the way to the modern virologists, investigators have only been able to acquire their knowledge from animals or from tissue cultures. During this time, hundreds of tumours were transplanted from one animal to another, and the Ehrlich carcinoma of the mouse and the Yoshida sarcoma of the rat had become the standard research material of science. But who could say that human and animal tumour cells would behave in absolutely the same way?

3,500,000 cancer cells in the arm

The prisoners in the Columbus penitentiary were not promised any privilege or remission of punishment. Nevertheless, within 24 hours almost a hundred of them reported to a provisional consulting room set up by Dr. Chester Southam of the New York Sloan-Kettering Institute. Under strict guard, each of them entered the room, laid bare his upper arm and was given an injection of 3½ million cancer cells.

With bated breath Southam and his colleagues watched what would now happen. In previous experiments the research team had found that cancer cells implanted into hopeless cases of cancer usually grew and multiplied for weeks or months, until they were ultimately removed. In these latest experiments, careful checks were made to see that none of the prisoners had been treated shortly beforehand by radiations or the adrenal hormone, cortisone. Treatment of this kind reduces the resistance of the body to implantations of foreign cells.

In a second series of experiments, normal cells were transmitted to cancer patients. This clearly showed that normal cells cannot grow in such circumstances. Cancer cells, on the other hand, actively increase. None of the patients showed a deficit of lymphocytes; each of them showed normal defence-reactions against bacteria and other stimulating substances, formed antibodies against viruses and were able to get rid of implanted normal cells. Why, then, could they not get rid of the implanted cancer cells? Was the reason to be found in the special properties of the cancer cells, or in the patients themselves?

Healthy people do not react

The experiment in the Ohio penitentiary gave the answer. The prisoners at first reacted with inflammation at the injection site. Then hard nodules appeared which went on growing for about two weeks. Examination under the microscope showed that these nodules were primarily composed of inflamed cells. The cancer cells, on the other hand, had become widely dispersed and showed all the signs of break-down.

After three weeks the nodules began to contract together: subsequently they all disappeared. None of them recurred.

Further studies were made on prisoners and cancer patients, which confirmed the previous observations. In the cancer patients, the implanted cancer cells were able to "gain a foothold" and to multiply. In the healthy prisoners, on the other hand, they were rejected completely. In these cases, too, no cancer cells remained after a few weeks: the defence mechanisms of the body had coped quite easily with them.

It was also found that patients with cancer that had not progressed far were also able to reject artificial cancer transplants. They reacted like the healthy prisoners. Their defence system against the transmitted cancer was thus sufficiently effective. Only when cancer was already far advanced did it appear that the defence mechanism no long functioned or was no longer intact.

This raised further questions. How would the respective subjects react to a second injection of cancer cells? As was to be expected, the response was both more prompt and stronger. The cancer cells grew more slowly in this second transmission, and disappeared much more quickly, than their predecessors. Even the prisoners first inoculated with only dead cancer cells, showed a stronger and more rapid defence reaction against living ones.

The results of these and subsequent tests suggested that there must be a common antigen which all cancer cells possess, but normal cells do not. New and refined methods of investigation showed that very few healthy people have such antibodies in their blood. Patients in whom the disease already existed, however, almost all possessed antibodies against transplants.

Still more detailed analyses showed that the rise and fall of the antibody level coincided with the growth and the subsequent rejection of the cancer cells. In addition, it was noted that in persons under investigation whose blood contained no antibodies, the cancer cells were rejected just as vigorously as they were in persons with plenty. This supported the view held by the research workers in the Sloan-Kettering Institute, that the chief part in the defence against tissue transplants is played by the antibodies constantly present in the cells and a smaller part by their variants circulating in the blood.

In healthy people under investigation i.e. in the volunteer prisoners, there was a stronger antibody defence against the cell type with which they were first inoculated. Between all the cancer cells used in the various experiments there were immunological cross reactions. On the other hand, there were none between the normal and the malignant cells. In none of the patients already suffering from cancer was it possible to detect antibodies against the cancer cells already present before the inoculations. "One thing emerges clearly from it all," said a summary by the Sloan-Kettering Institute, "The immunological defence present in healthy people, is absent in cancer patients under certain conditions. But we still do not know what the defect consists of."

Cancer cells a normal biological occurrence?

Do many people have a specific immunity to cancer? How does it happen that millions of cancer cells are frequently found in the blood streams of patients who have recently been operated upon, without these cells forming secondary tumours?

Science is so far unable to answer this question. Whilst many cancer investigators, (such as K. H. Bauer, for example,) flatly reject a special defence system against cancer cells, others are firmly convinced that malignant cells only become fatal if they are not recognised in time and killed by the immune systems of the body. As the German pathologist Christian Hackmann said: "The local formation of some abnormal cells is perhaps a normal biological occurrence which happens several times in the lifetime of every individual."

That these cells do not automatically lead to the formation of tumours is also the view of some of the greatest American authorities on cancer. Dr. Frank Horsfall, President and scientific Director of the Sloan-Kettering Institute, said: "Cancer cells can demonstrably be distinguished from normal cells. The normal organism can recognise them and can evoke immune reactions by which they are destroyed. Patients with advanced cancer have, under certain conditions, disorganised conditions of immunity."

Single cells can lead to a tumour – and thus to cancer. But they cannot do this if the defence system of the person affected is intact and functions adequately. If it does, the malignant cells die without that person knowing they have existed. Therefore cancer investigators and immunobiologists nowadays work in close collaboration, in order to learn more about the mysterious factors which permit or prevent, promote or inhibit, the unlimited growth of tissue.

Their work can sometimes have great significance. Professor Alexander Haddow, Director of the Chester Beatty Institute, admits that he looks to immunology and embryology for the next major advances in cancer research, and Dr. Horsfall of the Sloan-Kettering Institute says: "one of our chief aims is the development of suitable methods to remedy the inadequate immune defence of cancer patients."

The immunological barrier

But what does this "dynamic system", as it was called by Professor Otto Westphal, consist of?

Long before cancer investigators studied immunology, it was the bacteriologists who concerned themselves with human or animal defence systems against invading foreign substances or micro-organisms. They forged the now classical concept of antigens, whether these are related to bacteria, viruses or other invading substances. Thus antigen now means everything that a body perceives to be foreign to itself, and to which it reacts with a specific defence.

The body protects itself against such invaders by three "defensive ramparts". The skin is the first rough barrier. If this is overcome and a foreign particle, such as a bacillus, penetrates into the body, additional defensive forces are ready. In the blood there are the white blood corpuscles – fully formed cells which can move independently. Some of them are able actually to eat cells foreign to the body, such as bacteria, and to digest them; for this reason they are called *phagocytes*, i.e. cell-eaters. Other white blood cells cannot do this, but it is agreed that they secrete defensive substances against invading foreign cells.

If the "foreigners" have succeeded in overcoming even these controls and in getting out of the blood into the lymph, they there encounter the lymph glands. These are small organs which are found at certain intervals along the lymphatic vessels. Here again there are phagocytes which kill invaders.

If these measures do not succeed against a major invasion, an even more important protective mechanism comes into play. Specific cells of the organism make antibodies – proteins which belong to the gamma-globulin fraction of the serum albumin. These molecules "adapt" themselves accurately to the invading protein compounds, combine with them and, by altering their chemical nature, make them harmless.

Innumerable variations are possible in the molecular structure of the protein compounds which make up bacteria, viruses or cells. Each bacterial strain, each kind of virus and each type of foreign cell thus has its own antigenic code. In order to neutralise this, the antibodies formed by the organism must also be specific. If, for example, an antibody has been formed against influenza virus A, it works only against this kind of virus and not against any others.

But if the organism has once encountered a certain foreign body, has formed an antibody against it and has overcome its infection, then the molecular model of the invader is indelibly retained in its "memory". If a later infection of the same kind occurs, then the specific antibody is immediately produced in immense quantities. The disease no longer occurs. The organism has become immune.

The success of protective inoculations depends on these immunological reactions. A small, and therefore harmless amount, of a certain foreign protein, such as a bacterial toxin, is administered. Thereupon the organism produces the specific antibody and becomes immune to a fresh infection of the same kind, either permanently or at least for a long time. The British doctor Edward Jenner demonstrated the possibilities of such protective inoculations against smallpox in the eighteenth century.

Why skin transplants fail

The ability of the organism to make antibodies is a great help to doctors in their campaign against disease. On the other hand, intolerance of foreign protein also constitutes an almost insuperable hindrance to many forms of medical treatment, such as the transplantation of organs. If it is necessary, for example, to remove a kidney surgically, then it should be theoretically possible to implant the kidney of another person or even of an animal donor.

But in practice such transplants almost always prove to be failures, because the transplanted kidney constitutes for the new host organism a foreign protein, and therefore antibodies are formed by which it is rejected. Organ transplants without special difficulties are possible only in monozygotic twins. Their hereditary substance is absolutely identical and they therefore have the same immune code.

Because of these immunological barriers, blood transfusions from one person to another must be undertaken with special care. Each of the various human blood groups is characterised by the presence or absence of special antigens. If blood containing one of these antigens is given to a patient who possesses its natural antibodies, the blood corpuscles clump together because of the antigen-antibody reaction. This may often be fatal.

Among human antibodies, scientists have detected two different kinds. There are the humoral antibodies which are first formed in cells such as those of the bone marrow or the lymphatic glands and then discharged into the blood serum. They can be carried by the blood to wherever the corresponding foreign bodies have penetrated. But in addition to these mobile humoral antibodies, there are also stationary ones, situated on the surfaces of cells, like the antibodies against tubercle bacilli. These sessile antibodies seem to be responsible for unpleasant immunological incidents, but often the interaction between the invader and the antibody proceeds almost imperceptibly. The antibody can, in such cases, gain the upper hand so quickly and so completely that the person is hardly aware of the conflict in his body.

In this it is clearly always foreign body material to which the defensive forces react. But in cancer it is not a question of foreign materials penetrating the organism from the outside. It is rather a question of abnormal cells that already belong to the body. Is the defence system able to identify these cells also as foreign, and therefore hostile? Or does it tolerate them? The whole of cancer research in the field of immunology turns on the answer to this question.

According to the results of recent research, every cell has an antigen or the pattern of one – an unmistakeable hallmark like the stamp that indicates the quality of different eggs. Presumably these antigens are formed in the microsomes, and then are attached to the surface of the cells as distinctive chemical marks. The decisive question now is whether a cell changes this antigen pattern when it becomes malignant, and adopts another chemical distinguishing feature.

Is there a special cancer antigen?

Many scientists have in the past hoped to discover a specific cancer antigen in the cells of different tumours. The discovery of such a foreign molecule would imply a battle won in the campaign against cancer, since an intact immune system would, in the course of time, make antibodies against these foreign cells for long enough to kill them completely. There are cancer investigators who explain in this way the many reports of "spontaneous recoveries" from cancer.

If such a general cancer antigen were present in all the various kinds of malignant cells, then cancer would probably lose many of its terrors. Perhaps it would be possible to inoculate animals with cancer cells, and wait until sufficient antibody was produced in their serum. This animal serum could then be injected into human cancer patients, whose bodies produce insufficient antibodies against the disease. But even this hope has aroused strong doubts: the serum treatment of diseases such as diphtheria and tetanus relies on the relatively short-term administration of animal proteins. In cancer, on the other hand, prolonged treatment is to be expected and this would involve an increased risk of sensitisation to the foreign serum. It has not so far been proved whether antibodies are actually able to penetrate into the cell.

A tumour vaccine is tested

In 1962 the Swedish immunologist Dr. Bertil Björklund went so far as to test an anti-cancer vaccine on volunteers, and thereby provoked a storm in the public press.

Björklund's vaccine was composed of the so-called Hela-cells. These cells were first cultivated in tissue culture, then killed with a zinc salt, and finally they ground up so finely that only the cell walls remained. These cell walls were then irradiated with ultraviolet light, and were scrupulously examined for sterility and non-toxicity before they were injected into the volunteers.

Björklund was convinced that his procedure provided "relatively pure antigens". Although more than 100 people were inoculated with this vaccine, and Björklund carried out further extensive experiments, nothing definite was learned about its action on cancer. Björklund said that much further research will be needed to determine whether the vaccine contains active antigenic properties.

Björklund, however, is still convinced that the vaccine is harmless. "All the people we experimented on were between 60 and 70 years old," he reported in 1965 to the American Cancer Society. "If viruses actually cause cancer in man, it must be assumed that they are widely distributed and are picked up by many people. At their age most of the people we experimented on had been in contact for a long time with such viruses. Even if this were not so, their remaining life expectancy is too brief to allow the development of a tumour."

The time is not yet ripe

Björklund's researches must still be regarded as highly controversial. Most immunologists consider that the time is not yet ripe for experiments on man with anti-cancer vaccines. On the other hand experiments on animals are done to an ever increasing degree in order to gain more knowledge in this sphere of immunology.

Dr. Maurice Hilleman of the research division of the American drug firm, Merck, Sharp and Dohme, succeeded – like others before him – in successfully treating hamsters with an anti-tumour vaccine. Hilleman first infected newly-born hamsters with SV-40 virus, which usually causes tumours in these animals in 90–120 days; however, after 34–76 days Hilleman adminstered a vaccine obtained from irradiated tumour cells. The result was as definite as it was encouraging. The resistance of the animals to the tumour growth was increased three to seven times by the vaccine. If viruses should be discovered which also cause cancer in man, Hilleman sees equal possibilities. A suitable vaccine could have a preventative effect, as it does in polio or measles, and even in people already suffering from cancer successful treatment would be possible with a virus-antigen-vaccine.

Has each tumour its own specific antigen?

However, many adherents of an immunisation theory advise caution: they do not believe in a universal antigen common to all malignant cells. A whole series of research results indicate, on the contrary, that each kind of tumour has it specific antigen. Consequently there must be many antibodies against cancer cells, so that people would have to be immunised against hundreds of different cancer-antigens in order to become completely immune to cancer. To do that would be extremely difficult, even if it were fundamentally conceivable.

Professor Harry Norman Green, of the University of Leeds, established the fact that cancer cells often lack certain antigens, a concept of the origin of cancer that has often been noted. Green started from an old observation made by his colleague Professor Haddow of the Chester Beatty Institute in 1935. Haddow's work had been done on rats into which a very malignant sarcoma, the Jensen-sarcoma, had been injected. This sarcoma grew very rapidly and would have killed the animals in a few weeks had they not been given daily injections of certain polycyclic hydrocarbons. With these injections it was possible to prevent the growth of the sarcoma completely, or at least to slow it down appreciably.

The most effective of the hydrocarbons proved to be those with the most marked carcinogenic properties. As X-ray irradiation had already revealed, the paradox was that the substances that caused tumours were also able to prevent them.

The hydrocarbons only prevented the growth of tumours which had been transplanted into the animals. They were powerless against spontaneous tumours or tumours produced by treatment with chemicals. The idea consequently arose that carcinogenic compounds prevented the growth of the tumours by a definite immunological process. But why, asked Professor Green, were they not active against spontaneous or induced tumours? To find the answer to this, prolonged study of the relationship between the tumour and the host organism was necessary. The fact that malignant tumours can penetrate into neighbouring tissues and find footings in remote parts of the body, whilst healthy tissue remains within normal limits, had also to be investigated. Ultimately Green was convinced that the immunological factors which enable the body to keep normal tissue within bounds must be more or less absent from tumour cells. Only thus could these tumours spread themselves without limits. Every organism possesses three kinds of antigen: antigens which all members of a certain species possess, antigens which are present in all the cells of a certain individual, but are not characteristic of all members of a species: and finally antigens which are characteristic for a certain tissue or cell-type.

In the origin of cancer only the tissue-specific antigen can play a part, as Professor Green said in a conversation in the Cancer Institute of the University of Leeds. These tissue-specific antigens are presumably proteins on the cell surface; in his opinion, they are responsible for controlling the growth of the cell tissue.

If, when organs are injured or wounded, the tissue affected must regenerate by cell-division in order to replace the part destroyed, then influences acting on the tissue-specific antigens could let the tissue cells "know" when they have to stop dividing and multiplying. But if these antigens are absent, then the cancer cells divide further and further without regard to the surrounding tissue. In the same way it would be possible to understand why cancer cells separate from a lung tumour and can form metastases in completely different tissues of the body, for example in the brain.

Cause or result?

Is the loss of one or more tissue-specific antigens the result of the conversion of a normal into a malignant cell, or does the shortage of the antigen cause the change? In other words: is the loss of the antigen the cause or the result of cancer?

In the light of current knowledge, Green believed that in chemically-induced tumours it is the loss of antigen which allows the cell to become malignant. "If this is so," he concluded, "this is also probably true for all kinds of malignant growth."

Green referred to experiments with the azo dye "butter yellow" which causes cancer of the liver, but not of other tissues, in rats. If butter yellow is added to the rats' food, cancer of the liver appears after about nine months. The dye combines with the liver cells of the animals, but not with other kinds of cells. After about four weeks this combination reaches a maximum, and ultimately it declines again. The resultant tumour no longer contains butter yellow, nor does it absorb more if further doses are given.

The chemical compound is between the butter yellow and the tissue-specific antigens of the liver cells of the rat. If they are fed with the dye for about four weeks, its content in the liver cells declines. Therefore, Green suggested, no more antigen with which the dye could combine is then present. From all these facts he deduced that, in this instance, loss of antigen is the cause of the cancer. "The strength of the immunity theory," thought Green's pupil, Clayson, of the Cancer Research Institute in Leeds, "is that it takes into account all the facts of the cancer process." Thus, for example, it explains the appearances of metastases and the invasive behaviour of cancer cells without the need for any other hypothesis.

In addition, the fact that the cancer cells multiply extremely slowly in many tissues, but explosively in others, becomes understandable, for, after all, the tissue-specific antigens are lost at quite different speeds. It is equally clear how growth can be easily arrested in transplanted tumours but only with great difficulty in tumours that are spontaneous or induced. Transplanted tumours contain great quantities of tissue-specific antigens. Spontaneous and chemically induced tumours lack them.

But substantiative experiments are at present still not possible, and Green's ideas must, for the time being, remain speculative.

It is believed most chemical carcinogens react with tissue-specific antigens. The resulting compound is recognised by the reticulo-endothelial system as being foreign, and it responds by forming antibodies. In the resultant conflict, most of the cells which have reacted with the chemical carcinogen die, and the organism tries to replace them by extensive multiplication of the tissue constituents. Some of the cells whose proteins have combined with the chemical carcinogen still survive the antibody attack; these try to escape further immune reactions by means of reduced antigen marking.

With viruses, another mechanism of carcinogenesis must be imagined. Green assumed that viruses which penetrate into the nucleus of the cell upset the enzyme balance controlled there by the genes and prevent the synthesis of the tissue-specific antigens. But it is also possible that certain viruses *supplant* the tissue-specific antigens in the transformed cells. It could also be that the virus eliminates the enzyme responsible for the formation of these antigens.

The causation of cancer by means of ionizing rays has long been ascribed to direct changes in the nucleic acids. Perhaps – Green thought – certain cells thereby lose the ability to produce sufficient tissue-specific antigens. In cancer resulting from prolonged over-production of cells, a deficit of cell nutrients and building materials must be taken into account. Under these conditions a cell would no longer be able to produce tissue-specific antigens; the end result would then be the malignant cell.

Errors in cell division are corrected

The Australian immunologist and Nobel Prize Laureate Sir Frank Macfarlane Burnet also tended to the opinion that loss of antigens robbed the cancer cells of immunological control. But Burnet saw two other possibilities: cells normally responsible for the immunisation may be inhibited in their task, or the malignant cells may develop such a strong growth potential that they "ride roughshod over" all immunological controls. Burnet said that "if a carcinogenic process is to succeed, these controls must be eliminated".

Burnet saw immunity reactions in terms of biogenesis (the history of development). According to this they did not evolve in order to combat infections. Their primary importance lay, on the contrary, in protecting an individual or a species from the spread of its own abnormal cells.

In this Burnet started from the fact, established by most geneticists, that in the specific multiplication of the nucleic acids errors occur repeatedly in the composition of the new heredity structures. Thus mutations occur from time to time in both the body cells and the germ cells. It is not disputed that a malignant cell must be differentiated from the normal by changes in its hereditary substance. Therefore it can be assumed that, in every long-lived creature, cells with a cancerous potential are formed. In the human body, thousands of millions of cells divide daily.

Consequently a biological regulator must exist which untiringly prevents or corrects the errors which may occur in the DNA replication. Nature's "spelling mistakes" in the copying of the genetic code, the somatic mutations, are thus corrected. Only if such "corrections" fail, and the malignant cell structure minus its antigen marking is not recognised as being foreign, does further growth of the tumour cells occur.

The revolt of the antibodies

Although the organism is normally able to distinguish precisely between the "self" and the "not self", the ability to do this is often absent or becomes disordered. Newly-born creatures learn only gradually their "biological identity", and therefore react less strongly, or not at all, during their first weeks of life to foreign substances. In adults, too, the recognition system may suddenly cease to function, and antibodies can be formed against the organism's own tissues and organs. Such as organism, whose "steering wheel" has slipped out of its hands may, under certain conditions, reject parts of itself as if they were transplants. Although Paul Ehrlich was already working at the beginning of this century on the phenomenon of horror autotoxicus, the study of auto-antibodies made no special advances for decades. The idea that the person could form antibodies against himself was regarded as more suitable for a biological chamber of horrors than to hard-headed scientific categories of thought. It was also unthinkable that the antibodies, the bodyguards of humanity, should suddenly face about and attack their own organism.

"Today we know," said Professor Pierre Grabar, Director of the Institute for Cancer Research in Villejuif, near Paris, "that auto-antibodies are quite normal. We have thousands of examples of their existence." Professor Grabar was for years a leading authority in the field of protein investigation before he switched to the study of cancer immunology. "I would, however, never have accepted my present post, had I not been firmly convinced that immunological phenomena are involved in cancer."

The double rôle of immune factors

Grabar considered it to be possible that immune factors play a double part in the drama of cancer: that there are immune factors which enable the organism to defend itself against cancer cells and, at the same time, influences of immunity which favour the origin of cancer.

In contrast to many other scientists, Grabar believed that the immune reactions of the body are not primarily a defence mechanism against invading foreign substances. In his view they are part of a physiological system which removes decomposition products from the body. "How would these compounds otherwise disappear?" This theory, which invests the gamma globulins with the functions of transport workers, has met with opposition from almost all his colleagues engaged on immunity problems. "Nowadays, however, many of my theses have been widely accepted," said Grabar.

According to Grabar there are, at the start of the cancer process, important cell changes which may lead to necrosis and the death of cells. Disturbance which is, for example, caused by chemical substances, alters the antigen relationships of the cells. Antibodies against these cells are then formed which are clearly regarded by the body as foreign. It may even happen that the body forms antibodies against the nucleic acids of its own cells, so leading to deformations of these acids. But perhaps, if the nucleic acids multiply themselves, that part of the molecule which is impounded, as it were, by the auto-antibodies, is not re-created.

The "lead pencil" theory

With the help of a lead pencil, Grabar tried to illustrate this rather abstract process. "Suppose that this lead pencil corresponds to a nucleic acid molecule with its endless sequences. If, now, auto-antibodies are attached to this molecule" – Grabar covered up about a fifth of his lead pencil – "then a decisive part of the nucleic acid is altered. These changes are then transmitted by cell division to the descendants of the cell." According to this "pencil theory," as Grabar called it, cancer only occurs if a certain section of the nucleic acid is affected, the part which is responsible for growth control or for the rate of cell division. "My theory," Grabar went on, "can certainly not explain the origin of all kinds of cancer. Presumably it has no significance in cancer caused by viruses – even if it should be valid for certain malignant human diseases."

At any rate, Grabar has proved by experiments on animals that auto-antibodies can appear against necrotic cells. To do this, mice were treated with carbon tetrachloride. After some time destruction of cells occurred and auto-antibodies were formed. Because the animals were reared under sterile conditions, bacterial or virus influences could be excluded. In this connection one of Grabar's colleagues, Dr. Seligman, found antibodies against deoxyribonucleic acid in the serum of people suffering from Erythematoides. In this disease there are very malignant lesions of the face which are presumably due to auto-immunity.

"We also know today," Grabar said, "that in 80 per cent of all cancer patients there are auto-antibodies against the organ affected by the malignant process." The formation of such auto-antibodies is clearly not the inevitable consequence of cancer; it is perhaps only one of the possible results.

Do antibodies penetrate into the cell?

Meanwhile, in experiments on animals, auto-antibodies were found which can react with ribonucleic acid. Grabar therefore supposed that antibodies which react with nucleic acids cannot be strictly specific. Otherwise they would not enter into combination with acids of quite different origin. "On this an infinite amount of research work has still to be done," said Grabar. "In particular, we know too little about what happens when antibodies combine with antigenic constituents in the interior of the cell. Normal antibodies which react, for example, against bacteria, do not penetrate into the cell, but combine with the substances on the cell surface. That is a vast difference."

Many scientists doubt, in fact, that antibodies can actually penetrate into the interior of the cell. If they cannot, Grabar's theory is undoubtedly refuted. "There are also good grounds," said Grabar "for the idea that the spread of a tumour is associated with the fact that the normal mechanism for forming antibodies is not functioning properly."

It is not only babies and very old people who suffer from a dangerous deficit of antibodies. People at any stage of life may also lack them. There may be various reasons for this: the antibody system may be disordered or defective. The chemical forces which bind antibodies and antigens together may be too weak or unstable. There may be such an excess of invading antigens that the amount of antibody produced against them is simply not sufficient.

Such a deficiency may have various causes. Among them are faulty nutrition, a lack of certain vitamins, or disease due to general debility. But most carcinogenic substances have this sort of effect, and cause reduction of the antibodies and debility of the whole immunity system. Foremost among these are X-rays, and alkylating substances, such hydrocarbons as methylcholanthrene and urethane. By their use, the immunity reaction in animals can be reduced to a minimum, so that the transplantation of foreign tissue or even whole organs can usually succeed.

Attack on two fronts

Many scientists therefore ascribe to carcinogenic substances a double mode of action. On the one hand they produce proliferating and abnormal cells, and on the other they simultaneously suppress the immunity reactions which normally eliminate them.

This is a fascinating idea. It readily explains the origination of cancer by irradiation and chemical substances. And other facts support the hypothesis, for the causation of cancer in animals is most easily accomplished if they are very young or if their thymus gland has been removed.

That carcinogenic substances exhibit a bifrontal attack is shown in a rather different way. Methylcholanthrene prevents a certain strain of mice from forming antibodies; at the same time it causes leukaemia in the animals. But if, on the other hand, this standard carcinogen is administered to another strain, in which methylcholanthrene does not cause leukaemia, the antibodies are not suppressed. Irradiations also diminish the formation of antibodies in young mice and simultaneously cause leukaemia.

On the other hand there is also much to be said against this theory. "Many substances are, in fact, able to cause cancer and simultaneously to suppress the immunity reactions," wrote Dr. M. G. Berenbaum of St. Mary's Hospital in London, a specialist in immunology. "But the two do not always go together."

A number of chemical drugs similarly inhibit or disorganise the formation of antibodies and the rest of the immune processes, but they have no carcinogenic effect. This is especially true of the corticosteroids – of antimetabolites or of colchicine, which is a poison to cell division. The amount of the dose plays a part here, and in order to produce a tumour in animals much smaller doses are generally needed than those necessary to suppress the immune reactions.

To complicate the picture still further: against the theory of the bifrontal attack of chemical carcinogens can be set the fact that non-carcinogenic substances which suppress immune reactions generally slow down or even prevent the growth of the tumour. Typical examples of this are the corticosteroids, which are also used in the treatment of cancer.

Finally it must also be mentioned that many malignant cells induced by chemical substances are from the start so vigorous and so insensitive to immune reactions that they break through all barriers. As Berenbaum wrote: "the ability to suppress all immunity processes might therefore be as unnecessary as it is inadequate to explain the origin of cancer."

A granule on the scales

He emphasized that investigation of the relationship between immunological processes and the origin of cancer is still in its infancy.

Final conclusions in this field, therefore, can still not be drawn. Thus, for example, the possibility cannot be excluded that small doses of carcinogenic substances cause a chronic subnormal functioning of the immune system, which is quite difficult to detect. But under certain conditions they have a critical effect on the early stages of the origin of cancer, and represent the granules which turn the scales in favour of the disease.

It should not be overlooked that most substances which inhibit immune reactions are standard preparations for cancer therapy. Experimental and clinical tests must therefore determine in which cases the use of these drugs is more injurious than useful.

The search for a specific cancer antigen proceeds independently with greater intensity. Many scientists, not only in the Western world, but also in the Soviet Union, hope to find such an antigen.

"Much is still not clear," wrote Dr. Lev Zilber of the Gamaleya Institute of Epidemiology and Microbiology in Moscow "but there is little doubt that a tumour-immunity actually exists. Our chief problem is to isolate and concentrate corresponding antigens. Possibly, once this task is completed, clinicians will be given the preparations which can be used for the diagnosis, prophylaxis and treatment of tumours."

A question of time?

Dr. Lloyd Old of the Sloan-Kettering Institute adopts a similarly optimistic attitude. For the last five years ("practically since immunological investigation in this field began") Old has also specialised in the discovery of cancer antigens. "Previously" he says "such cancer antigens were merely a vague hope, a wishful dream of many scientists. Now we already know such antigens exist in animals. Clearly they must be detected in man." In Old's opinion it is extremely improbable that such specific antigens are not present in human tumours. "Their discovery is probably only a matter of time."

The discovery of tumour-specific antigens in animals has, in Old's words, revealed "the first qualitative difference between healthy and malignant cells. Clearly the hope that it will be possible to find the same antigen in all kinds of cancer must definitely be abandoned."

Tumours caused by the same virus always contain the same characteristic cell-antigen. Tumours caused by chemical carcinogens, on the other hand, show different antigens, even if they are caused by the same carcinogen. In the Sloan-Kettering Institute the same chemical carcinogen has simultaneously induced different tumours in different parts of the body of a single mouse, and these contained different antigens. "That is indeed the strongest evidence that can be brought against the theory of a universal cancer antigen."

Where do the cancer antigens in the tumours come from? In chemically-induced tumours – which seem to be especially rich in antigen – the carcinogen itself may well not have any antigenic properties. It is possible that the antigens are products of altered genes. But they may also represent normal parts of genes which remain suppressed in differentiated cells and are only set free by malignant processes in the interior of the cell.

With viruses it is conceivable that an antigenic constituent takes over the new immunological "marking" of the malignant cells. The virus would then be responsible for the ability of these cells to develop a transplantation-immunity. Since infectious viruses are constantly found in transplanted virus leukaemia, it is very difficult to determine what the specific antigenic property is to be ascribed to. It could arise if virus material were incorporated in the cell membrane, or if new cell-antigens were formed. These cell antigens would then be controlled either by the DNA of the virus or by that of the transformed cells.

Flooding with tumour cells

Although in Polyoma-tumours the virus can no longer be detected, a definite antigen remains. Old sees here evidence of a new cell-antigen which is independent of the virus. There is direct proof that genetic material of the virus is incorporated in other virus tumours. Such proof would also exist when the virus can no longer be isolated. According to Old, cancer must be ascribed in every case to a defective immunity system. "We have, in our experiments on animals, always observed that tumours grow intensively in spite of very strong immune reactions." Probably in such cases the immune system is simply overwhelmed. In mice, tumours induced by chemical carcinogens were successfully transplanted by inoculations of only 40 cells.

If, for example, about four million cells are inoculated, a tumour develops. This number of malignant cells is too great for the defensive forces. But with only 40 cells the amount of antigen is so small that it escapes detection, and these cells can likewise develop. Especially if the injection site is far removed from the places where the organism develops its immune reactions. With advanced development and the corresponding amount of antigen it is then too late.

If animals are inoculated with about 40,000 cells the chances of resistance are best – there is then enough antigen present to excite a defence reaction, but the attack is not so strong that it can overrun the defences.

If there is no universal cancer antigen, does this mean that all hope of a vaccine is lost? Old does not think so. "We can start from the fact that there is not an unlimited number of such antigens. Perhaps there are no more than 30 to 50. Thus a kind of polyvalent vaccine against most kinds of cancer can be conceived."

Meanwhile there are other problems for Old to solve. Where, for example, are cancer antigens situated and what is their chemical nature? There is much evidence that these antigens are to be found in the cell membrane. But the Hungarian Immunologist George Klein, who now works at the Karolinska Institute in Stockholm, has yet another hope. To the IXth International Congress on the Study of Cancer in Tokyo he said that probably all kinds of cancer pass through a common stage. If this is so it must be possible to find a remedy that is equally effective at this stage in every type of cancer.

Increase of the natural defences

Not less important and perhaps less difficult to solve is the problem of non-specific resistance. This is a matter of the attempt to strengthen the natural resistance of the body by immune reactions. It should be possible to increase considerably the production of antibodies and lymphocytes by chemical or biological means. This would be a tempting possibility not only in cancer but also in many other diseases. Recent investigations have shown that the antibodies bound to the protein constituents of the blood are much less active against cancer cells than are the antibodies coupled with the white blood cells, especially with the lymphocytes produced by the thymus gland.

Science for many years "looked down its nose" at this small organ, which in man lies just behind the upper part of the sternum and weighs only 10–20 grammes. It was considered to be a quite insignificant part of the lymphoid system, i.e. those organs which include the bone marrow, the spleen and the lymph glands.

The actual function of the thymus was for a long time not clearly established. Its investigation seemed hardly worth while, if, as was thought, it was a useless gland which in man underwent involution and disappeared after the 20th year of life.

Three investigations suddenly drew experts' attention to this "Cinderella" gland. If, for example, the thymus was removed from new-born hamsters, the animals suddenly became susceptible to a virus that had been found in human cancer cells. If the thymus of mice was destroyed by X-rays, the animals developed leukaemia. If the thymus was removed from new-born-rabbits, they lost weight, sickened and died.

Many experiments on other animals have since shown that the thymus is one of the most important of organs. It seems to act as a master organ of the lymphocytes and antibodies, and therefore of a large part of the whole immune system. "Probably," said Professor Bernhard Halpern of the Collège de France, who has won world-wide fame as an investigator of allergy, "the thymus gland is the origin of the mysterious mechanisms which determine the recognition of 'self' and 'not-self' and all the other immunological processes."

The Canadian Dr. J. A. F. P. Miller, and Dr. Robert Good of the University of Minnesota, have recently been distinguished by their studies of the thymus. They have found that after removal of the thymus, the blood of new-born animals contains very small quantities of antibodies. Tissue transplants from one animal to another are therefore especially easy. Clearly there are not enough antibodies present to reject the foreign tissue.

Do viruses weaken the thymus?

According to Dr. Robert Good, the thymus is the first of all the immunity organs of the unborn creature to develop during pregnancy. From it, the first cells migrate to the different parts of the body; to the lymph glands, the tonsils and to the appendix (caecum). They thus lay down the foundation of the lymphoid tissue, including the lymphocytes. Good postulates that there is in at least one kind of cancer, namely, acute leukaemia in early childhood, a relationship to the thymus. Thus perhaps viruses could weaken the thymus gland; this would prevent lymphocytes from being mobilised for the protection of the body against leukaemia.

This theory is, for the time being, quite vague. The distinctive part played by the lymphocytes as police forces in the human body is clearly no longer contested, so the question was posed: could the production of these blood cells, which are so important to life, be artificially stimulated, or could lymphocytes be supplied to the body from the outside, if the body itself could no longer produce enough of them?

There had already been numerous attempts at such a transfusion of lymphocytes. They showed that lymphocytes can, in fact, be transferred from one organism to others. In contrast to the transference of foreign blood or protein substances, this did not cause unpleasant defence reactions. The lymphocytes must, however, be taken from the lymph system before they circulate in the blood stream.

Peter Alexander of the Chester Beatty Institute has special experience in relation to lymphocytes. He took parts of tumours which had been induced in rats and transplanted pieces of them into rats of other strains. From animals in which these tumours did not develop, lymphocytes were taken after about a week and injected into rats with tumours. After theses injections, the tumours actually degenerated. But lymphocytes from animals which had not previously been immunised by transplanted tumour cells showed no effect when they were inoculated. The tumours in the animals remained unaffected and continued to grow.

Further investigations were clearly disappointing. Unfortunately by no means all lymphocytes could be "specialised" in such a manner for the campaign against cancer cells. Only a hundredfold excess of lymphocytes derived from animals immune to tumours could destroy a single individual cancer cell. Many tumours consist of thousands of millions of cancer cells. Astronomical numbers of lymphocytes would therefore have to be assembled and injected.

An indicator of immunity?

Immunological control of cancer still has a long way to go, and no one can yet judge what significance it will have. Certainly the climax of all immunological research would be a cancer vaccine which would prevent the outbreak of the disease, or would bring about the involution of tumours that already exist.

Even an investigator as obsessed with the subject as Dr. Chester Southam of the Sloan-Kettering Institute, who dared to carry out the experiments in the Ohio penitentiary, at present ascribes only a relatively limited place to immunological methods. However, Southam advanced to the Congress of the American Cancer Society in 1965 three theses, the clarity of which leaves nothing to be desired.

1. Man has a natural immunity against cancer;

Ten thousand chemical substances are tested annually in laboratories for their effects against cancer. Professor Hans Lettré (above) and Professor Hermann Druckrey (below) are two cancer research workers of international fame.

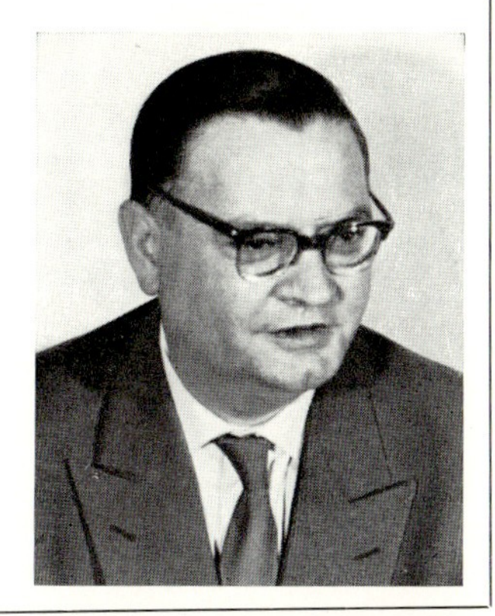

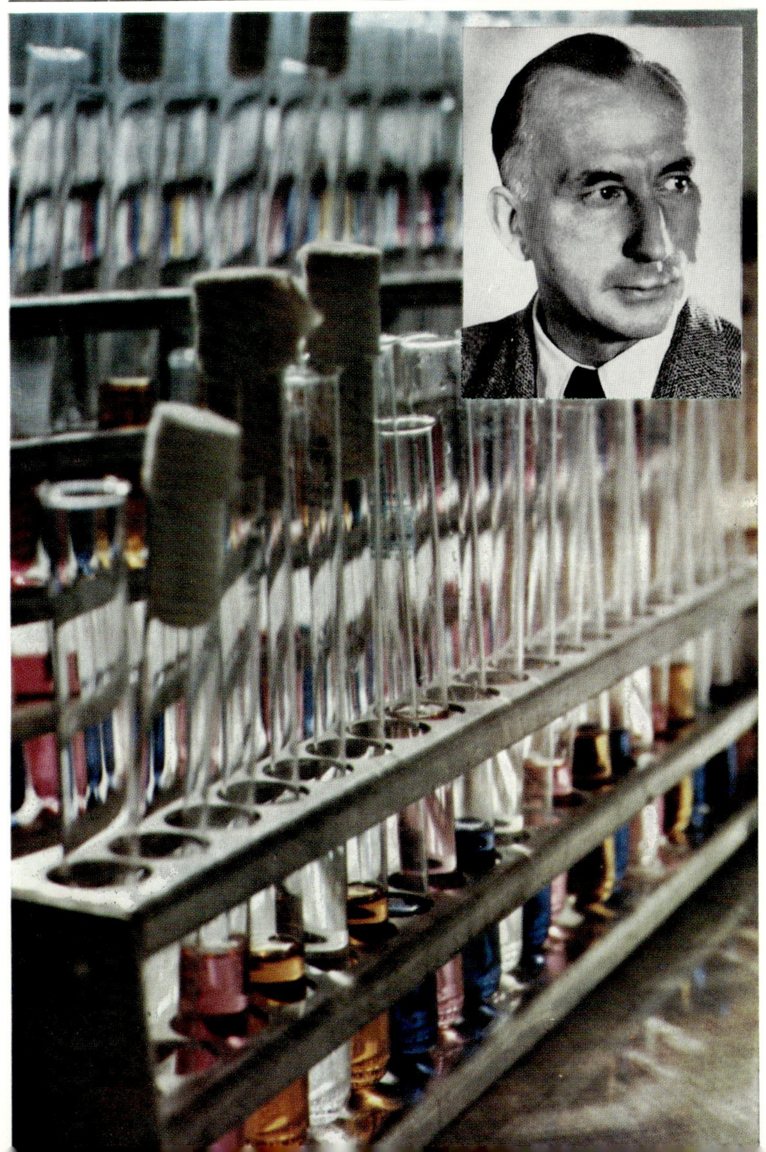

Much outstanding research has been done on carcinogenesis in the Chester Beatty Institute in London. Its Director is Sir Alexander Haddow.

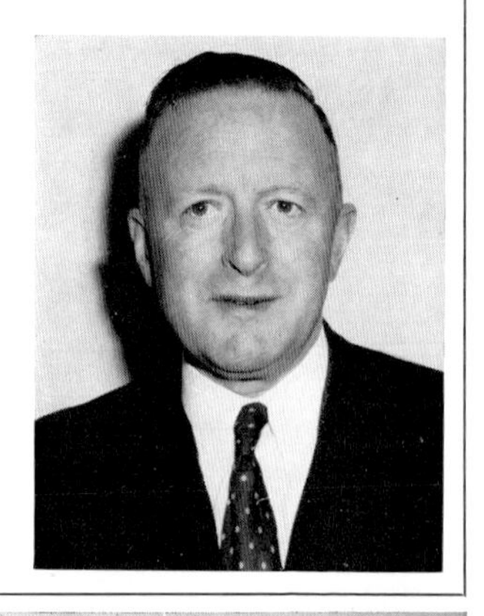

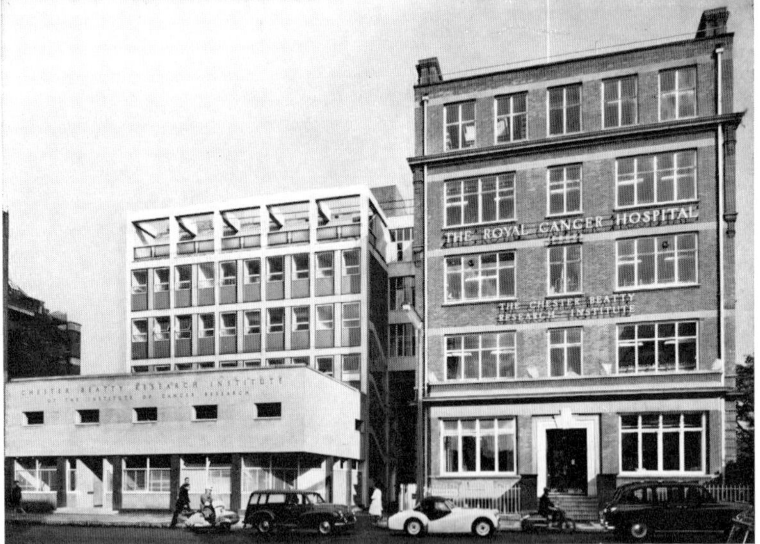

Part of the apparatus for the manufacture of the chemotherapeutic substance, "TEM", at Farbwerke Hoeschst A.G.

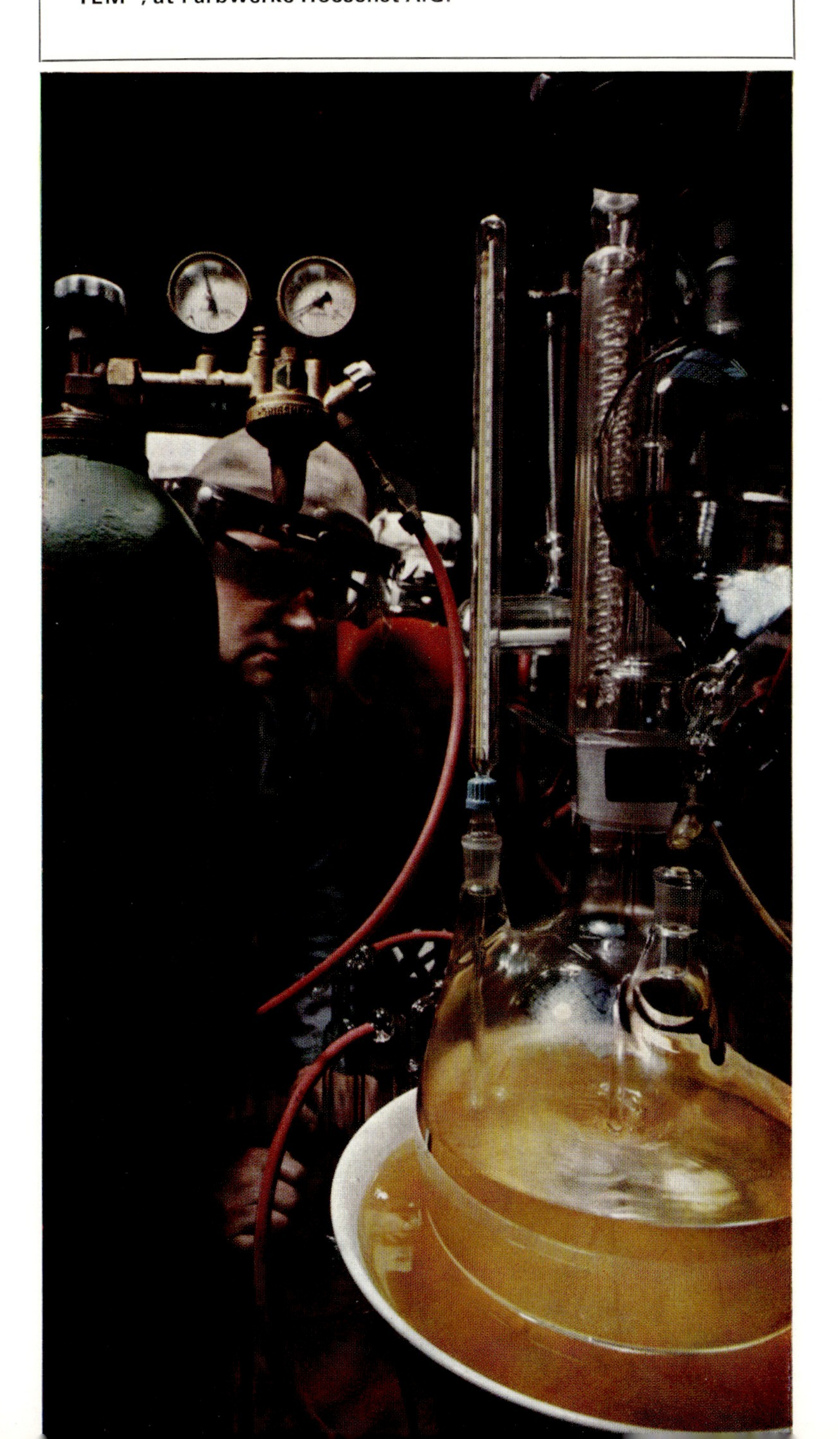

Previously, tumours could only be maintained by transplantation from one animal to another. Nowadays tumour tissue can be preserved for a long time in special tumour banks.

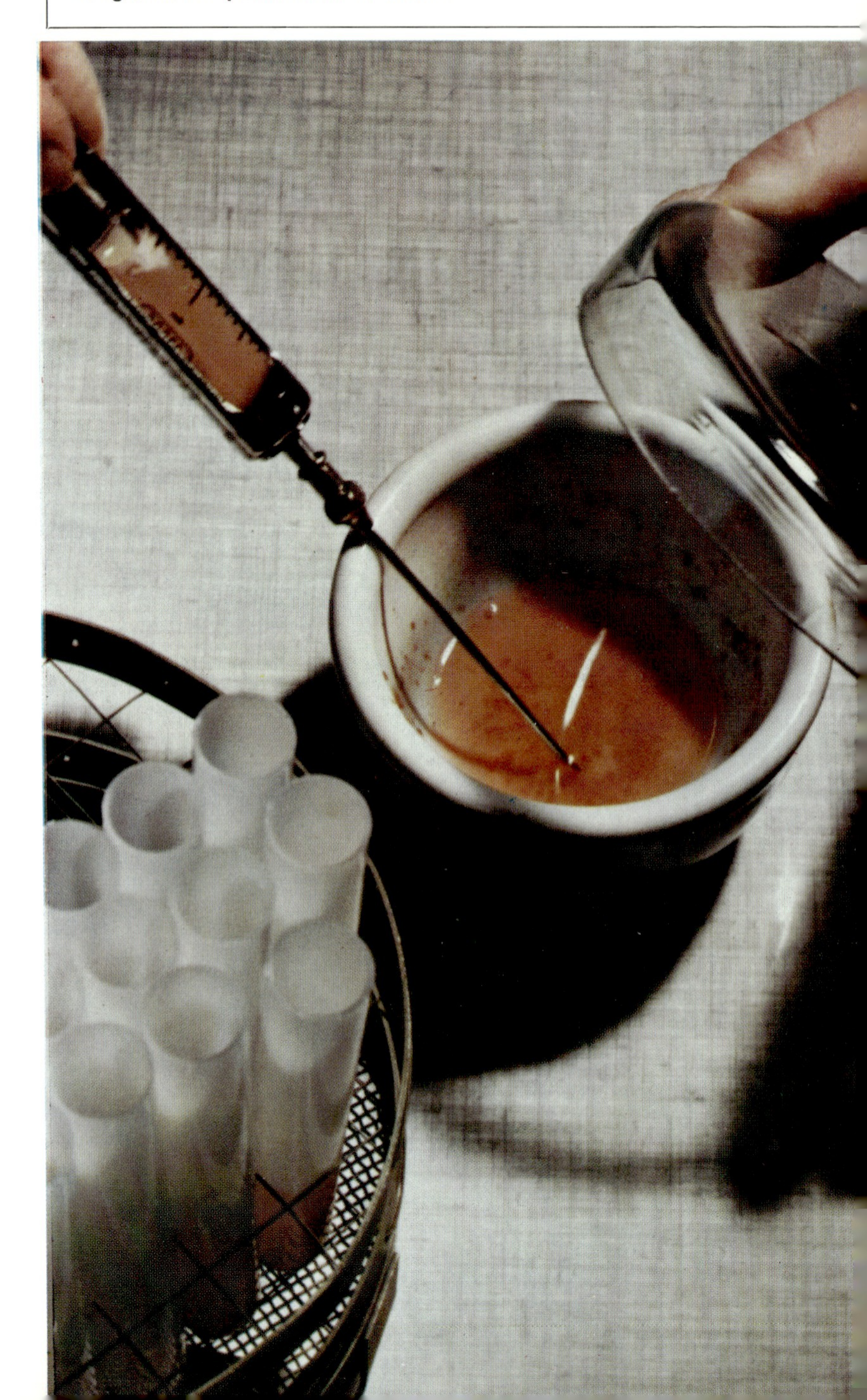

e tissue is macerated. After the
lition of preservatives (shown in
picture on the left) the cellular
terial is frozen (see the picture on
right) with liquid nitrogen at a
nperature of −196 C.

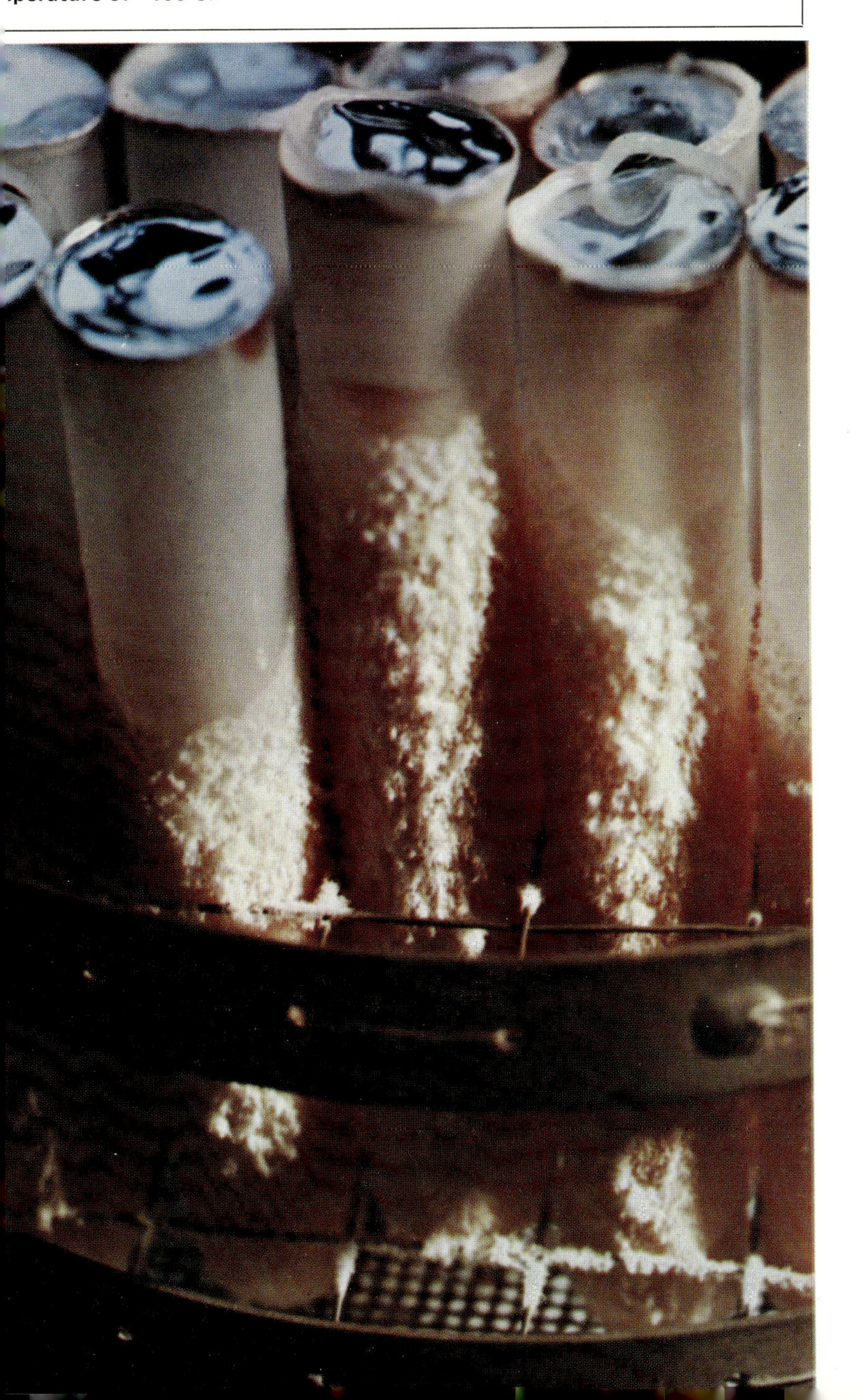

Cells of a Yoshida sarcoma of the rat. This tumour belongs to the standard strain used internationally. It bears the name of the Japanese cancer research worker, Professor Tomizo Yoshida, President of the 9th International Cancer Congress held in Tokio, in October 1966.

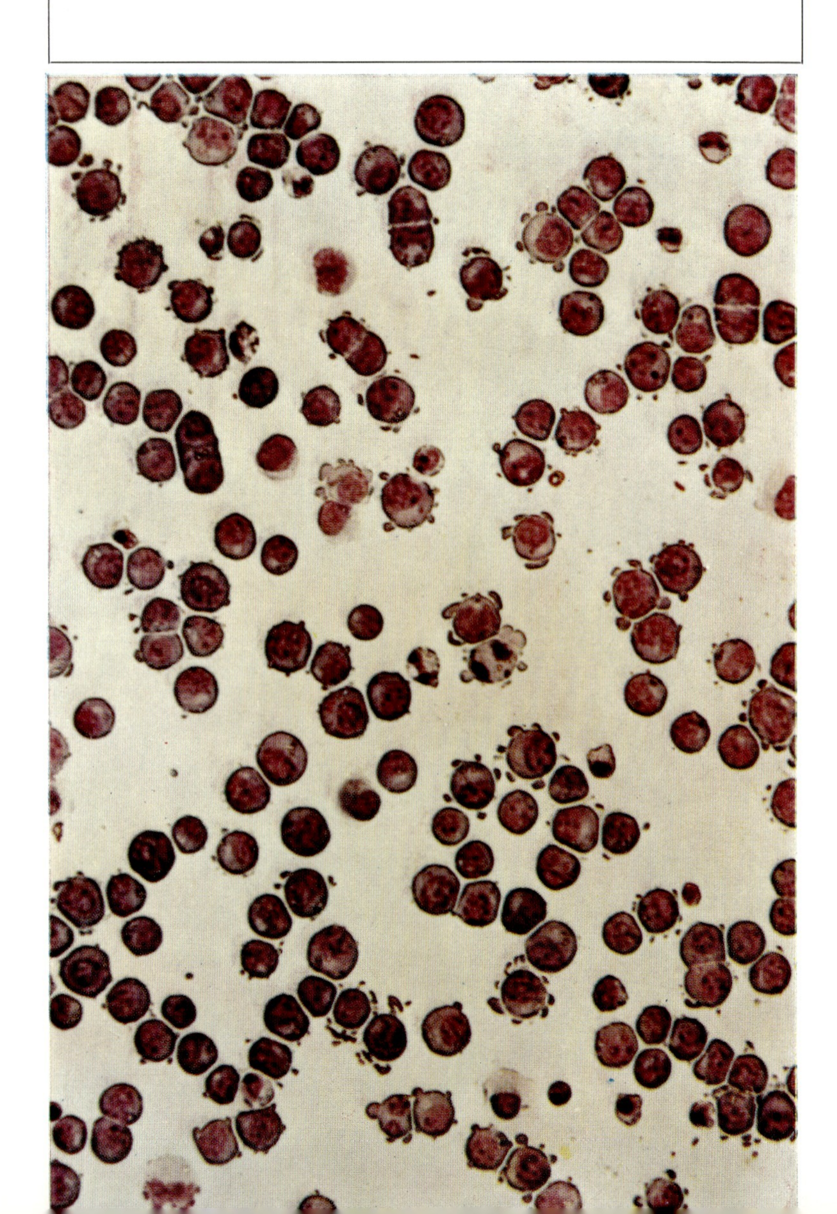

Two distinguished French cancer investigators: Professor Pierre Grabar (top), Director of the Institute of Cancer Research in Villejuif, near Paris, and Professor Georges Matthé (bottom) of the Institute of Cancer and Immunogenetics (shown in the middle picture).

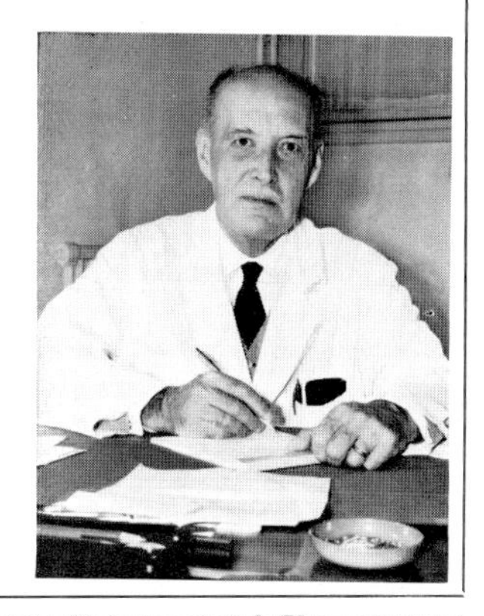

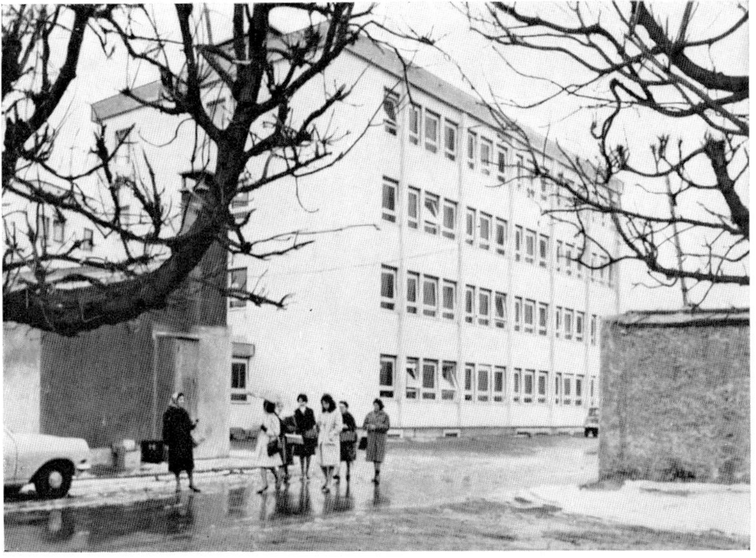

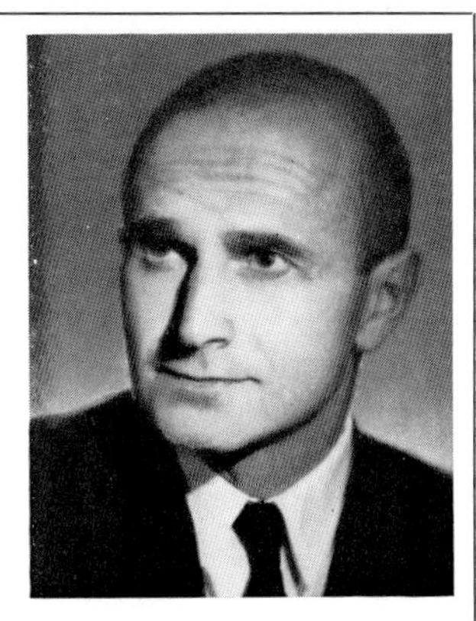

Professor Wilhelm Flaskamp, President of the North Rhineland Westphalian Society for Combating Cancerous Diseases, played an influential part in the establishment of a cancer research institute in Essen.

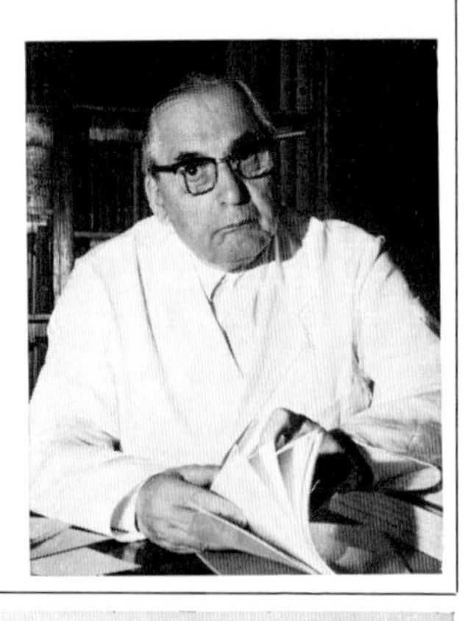

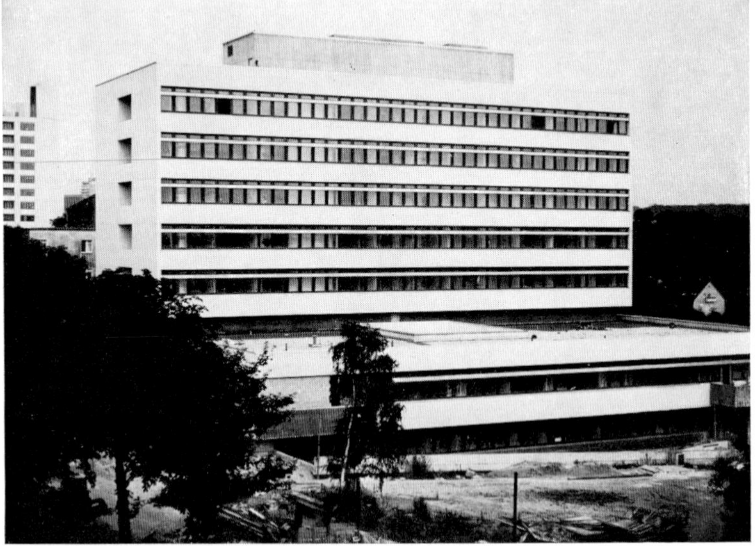

2. People suffering from cancer have a weakened immunity to the disease.

3. It is possible to measure the degree of the weakness of immunity in a cancer patient.

The immunological relationships in cancer patients can be determined to a certain degree by means of the serum-protein component properdin, which was found in the blood some years ago and seems to provide a relatively good criterion for assessing the defensive forces of the body.

According to researches so far done, properdin is able, at any rate in nocturnal haematuria, to break down the pathologically altered red blood corpuscles. It is, however, very doubtful whether it can have this effect on tumour cells. For cancer investigators claim to have found that in many cancer patients with a normal properdin level, the disease proceeds considerably better than in patients with a very low properdin content in their blood.

Investigations in the sphere of immunity must probably continue for many years. According to Southam it will one day be possible to eradicate, by immunological methods, the last nests of cancer cells remaining in the body after surgery. irradiation or treatment with drugs.

Southam's most recent experiments were done in the James Ewing Hospital and the Memorial Hospital of the Sloan-Kettering Institute. These lasted for three years. Southam injected two different preparations into patients with very advanced cancer. The first contained cancer cells taken from the patients's own tumours. The other came from the normal tissues of healthy persons.

These experiments showed that cancer patients in general do not reject transplants of their own tumours into other parts of the body. Occasionally they have not even the power to reject normal tissue. In this Southam saw the chief proof that the normal body defence no longer functions sufficiently.

Excess of antigens

Dr. Jacob Furth of Columbia University has also referred to this insufficient defence in a weakened organism. He found that the cell changes caused by carcinogenic chemicals, viruses, irradiation or other agencies, also always have an additional effect: the cells that have now become malignant produce new antigens.

"Unfortunately," Furth explained, "the malignant cells produce more antigens than the weakened body can render harmless by means of antibodies." It is only this excess of antigens that then permits the cancer cells to develop unrestrictedly.

Dr. Furth put forward these ideas in a lecture at which a young medical student of the Wayne State University was present. To this student, Norbert Czajkowski, the inference was as clear as it was to his fellow-students: a way must be found to mobilise and strengthen the defensive forces of the organism threatened by cancer.

The result was that an immunological technique occurred to him which had already been developed decades earlier. Not all foreign substances act as antigens. It is only foreign proteins that exert a sure antigenic action. These proteins are immediately recognised by the body as being foreign and are resisted by means of antibodies. In experiments on animals, immunologists had therefore studied what happens if non-antigenic substances are combined with foreign proteins, and this new compound is introduced into the body.

Immunity by means of aspirin

The result was startling: the organism produced antibodies against the protein fraction of the compound administered. But it also developed antibodies against the substance combined with it which normally, if administered alone, caused no immunological reaction. It was thus possible to provoke an immune reaction against even as simple a substance as aspirin.

What would happen, reflected Czajkowski, if this technique should be also used in cancer? He took malignant tissue from mice suffering from tumours and bound to it a foreign protein, namely, human gamma globulin. Then he injected it again into the same mice. And in fact the method worked. He found that the mice now actually developed antibodies against their own cancer cells. But what was still more important the tumours underwent distinct involution.

After a year of experiments on 34 mice, the method was also used on 20 human patients who voluntarily made themselves available. All other kinds of cancer treatment had shown themselves to be unsuccessful.

First of all, tumour tissue was removed from the patients and pulverised. Further "ingredients" were gamma-globulin from rabbits, which always has an antigenic effect in the human body, and a chemical reagent which brings about a combination between the gamma globulin and the tumour tissue. Finally yet another chemical substance which helps quite general immune reactions, was added to this mixture of substances. The new preparation was then injected into the patients.

Of the 20 patients who were considered as certain candidates for death, two women were alive and free from tumours 3½–4 years later. In eight other patients the tumours had largely undergone involution. The remainder could not be saved.

Dr. Czajkowski – he has meanwhile completed his medical studies – is extremely cautious. He emphatically declared that "the results of our research do not justify any hope of a cancer cure that is speedy and superior to all other methods. At present we have only an interesting experimental technique. It is still not by any means near the stage which insulin treatment, for example, had reached when Banting and Best produced their first publications."

A long programme of additional research is in store for Czajkowski. First, the point of the tumour cells at which the antigen is formed has to be accurately located. Then it is necessary to elucidate the biochemical structure of this antigen. And finally, chemical substances and foreign proteins have to be sought, which were more active than those used in the first research. At least two further years and considerable financial resources are required before success in these researches can be expected, says Czajkowski. At the same time he hopes that work will be done on his method in the future at other research centres. "Perhaps then advances can be accelerated."

Exchange of tumour tissue

In the Roswell Park Memorial Hospital in Buffalo, another method of immunisation is being tested. Groups of patients were formed each consisting of two patients with tumours of a similar size. Into each of the two patients, tumour tissue from the "partner" was transplanted. After a certain time this foreign tissue was rejected by the organism, but not before antibodies against the foreign tissue had already been formed. Finally, cross transfusions of white blood corpuscles were undertaken between the two patients. A total of 26 persons took part in this research. In two patients complete involution of the cancer was observed, and in 5 others a partial involution. This was particularly true of melanomas.

Among the white blood corpuscles, the lymphocytes will play the chief part in future immunological treatment of cancer, Dr. Furth expects. He points out that many cancer antigens are to be found in the lymphocytes, but not in the blood serum. "An enormous advance towards the clinical control of malignant tumours" would occur, in Dr. Furth's opinion, "if such lymphocytes could successfully be cultivated outside the body and then 'trained' to attack the specific cancer antigens". In the treatment as large a part of the tumour as possible must first be surgically removed. From it a vaccine would be prepared. At the same time, the tumour antigens would be given to lymph cells of the patient cultivated outside his body. When the lymphocytes had been thus "trained" to the tumour antigens, they would again be injected into the patient.

Prevention rather than treatment

However, this vision of the future founders for the time being on a particular obstacle: the technique of the tissue culture of lymphocytes *in vitro* has not advanced so far that it would be possible to cultivate these cells in the large quantities required for such a procedure. Immunologists clearly hope for more from a preventive inoculation than from cancer treatment. Dr. David W. Weiss Berkeley has injected suspensions of tumour tissue from mice suffering from mammary carcinoma into normal young adult mice. He has achieved in this way an immunity against later transmissions of the same tumour. The cells of this form of cancer, which is caused by a virus, develop, so Weiss postulated, two antigens – an antigen of the virus itself and another, independent of the virus, which is probably produced by the conversion of the cells into their malignant form.

It goes without saying that in virus cancer the outlook for immunological control would be especially favourable. So far, as has been stated, virus cancer has been discovered only in some species of animals. If it should one day be identified in types of human cancer, for example, forms of leukaemia, immunology would certainly be given a stronger stimulus.

In the United States work is proceeding on a vaccine for the prevention of leukaemia. Some large pharmaceutical firms have already made trial quantities of such a vaccine. But no one can say whether they will be effective.

Accurate weapons against malignant cells

Although immunologists may face a long, hard road, they provide the greatest hope in the campaign against cancer. Professor Alexander Haddow, who revealed that he expected the greatest advances to occur in the immunological field, is not alone in this opinion. Surgeons and radiologists have probably reached the highest point of their art, and in chemotherapy a decisive success will only be possible if a drug is developed which selectively kills cancer cells.

Immunotherapy, on the other hand, could develop into an unerring weapon against cancer cells, without injury to the healthy organism. This would not only be treatment after the event; it would offer the positive chance of preventing cancer. If one day the time should come when inoculations against cancer are as common as they now are against smallpox, infantile paralysis or measles, then the disease could become equally rare.

Many research workers regard such an idea as wishful thinking; others firmly believe in its possibility. But there are many problems still to be solved, especially the crucial ones of whether cancer cells differ immunologically from healthy cells, and whether the defensive forces of the body can ultimately be stimulated and activated sufficiently to suppress a major cell revolt.

For the surgeon who seeks to replace damaged organs and tissues by means of transplants, the immunological defences against foreign tissue are a great obstacle. He must try in every way to overcome them.

Cancer therapy on the other hand, demands exactly the opposite. Immunologists must strengthen the specific defence of the body, so that it recognises not only foreign substances and tissues as antigens, but even its own cells, whose anarchy has become a threat to life.

Although immunological research has still not succeeded in making a radical break-through in the campaign against cancer, it has already made valuable contributions to cancer theory. It is no longer possible to believe simply that cancer begins with the conversion of a normal body cell into a cancer cell and that all the rest follows automatically if this damaged cell multiplies itself further. Many factors must combine to favour the growth of a malignant cell into a tumour which can be regarded as "cancer."

There is a great chance

This clearly indicates that cancer is not a general affliction and the tumour only an obvious symptom. Opinions are nowadays varied. Some investigators think that cancer may be a local disease, others consider it to be a general one. Probably it can be both. It is therefore important to find, among the numerous possibilities, the right starting point for treatment. There is a great chance that immunology will provide this.

Chapter 9

PREVENTION – BETTER THAN CURE

Chemotherapy and immunology – these are the two weapons, without doubt, with which mankind will seek to ward off the relentless enemy. But when will it not only be possible to prolong the lives of cancer patients, but also to save most of them. An agonisingly long time will doubtless pass before that happens. Far too long for millions of people for whom the result of the research campaign will come too late.

Many investigators believe that the final triumph over cancer will only be possible when the "extremely delicate" biochemical difference which exist between normal and malignant cells can be determined. Only when the mysterious growth of cancer cells and the action of carcinogenic substances can be completely explained will it be possible to find certain methods of killing malignant cells or of returning them to the control systems of the body.

The dramatic history of medicine clearly proves that it has so far been possible successfully to control or check diseases without elucidating their ultimate causes. In a series of diseases, such as diabetes, no cause has been definitely explained. Nevertheless, they are now completely controlled by drugs. Medicine is indebted to happy accidents by research workers, or to sheer intuition, for many of the modern "wonder-drugs".

In cancer, too, further and perhaps even decisive chemotherapeutic achievements are conceivable without need for detailed explanation of the biochemical process of cell damage, or even of the processes in the healthy cell with its millions of molecules.

Moreover, famous investigators do not expect that cancer will only be overcome by treatment. It may be still more promising to prevent its occurence. Without doubt, in the future, immunological methods and anti-cancer vaccines will play an important part, whether against cancer caused by chemical substances or by viruses. The virologist Dr. Bernice Eddy thinks that "cancer, like every infectious disease, may be more easily prevented than cured".

She thinks that the outlook for an effective vaccine against oncogenic viruses depends on whether further research shows that only a restricted number of viruses can cause cancer. In this case, it will be necessary to render the carcinogenic part of the virus, the nucleic acid, completely harmless.

Clearly, as has already been pointed out, by no means all cancer investigators consider the existence of specific cancer antigens in man to be proved, or even probable. But there is still agreement that methods must be found to strengthen the preparedness of the body for defence. In America, much work has been done on such "boosters of immunity" for the prophylaxis of cancer, particularly since the impression has gained ground that many forms of leukaemia, and of other cancerous diseases, can be ascribed to virus infections. According to this, the malignant process only begins when the defence forces of the body have been broken down.

Anticarcinogens: a great hope

Some time ago a new ray of hope emerged, namely, the possibility of immunising man against chemical carcinogens – one of the most exciting prospects in cancer research. This involves the so-called anti-carcinogens which act as rivals of the carcinogens. Benzpyrene and dibenzanthracene, two highly-active carcinogens, almost completely lose their effect when experimental animals are injected with compounds that are chemically very similar to them. Clearly this is a question of the concurrence of two chemical substances, in which the carcinogen in the cell is neutralised by another compound which is either non-carcinogenic or only a weak carcinogen.

Two research workers in the American National Cancer Institute, Hans L. Falk and Paul Kotin, have tested such anticarcinogens in extensive experiments on animals. First of all they used three compounds closely related to the carcinogenic hydrocarbon dibenzanthracene. In each case, 30 microgrammes of the carcinogen and fifteen times as much of one of the anticarcinogens were simultaneously injected subcutaneously into thirty mice. It was found that two of the anticarcinogens were able completely to suppress the formation of tumours. In animals which had received only the carcinogen, but not the anticarcinogen, tumours developed 4–7 months after the injection.

The two American scientists obtained a quite similar effect with methylcholanthrene, which is very strongly carcinogenic, and with three non-carcinogenic compounds closely related to it. Here, also, fifteen times as much anticarcinogen as methylcholanthrene was administered simultaneously, and the development of tumours was suppressed.

The effect of the respective anticarcinogens would clearly be considerably affected by the solvent used for the carcinogen and the chemical substances associated with it. The time factor also revealed great differences in the effect on tumour growth. With dibenzanthracene as the carcinogen and phenanthrene as the anticarcinogen, the inhibition of tumour growth was most marked when the two substances were injected either simultaneously or at an interval of not more than two days.

The greater the time interval, the weaker was the effect on the tumour growth. Still more interesting were experiments in which benzpyrene was used as the carcinogen. It is known that this is a carcinogen frequently encountered in man's environment, whether in cigarette smoke, dust, impure air, or foodstuffs.

Falk and Kotin wished to find out whether the effect of the carcinogen is influenced by other widely distributed substances which do not cause cancer. For this purpose they used mixtures of polluted air collected in different States of America. These studies lasted 17 months. They showed that various compounds present in the filtered air mixture had an inhibitory effect on the carcinogenic activity of benzpyrene.

The forces of the chemical antagonists

Clearly, at present, the whole mode of action of the carcinogenic hydrocarbons is not completely known. In each case a considerable excess of anticarcinogens must be mustered in order to prevent cancer being caused by the carcinogenic substances. A competitive inhibitory effect is clearly still most likely.

But presumably further extensive research on how carcinogens and anticarcinogens act in the cell will very soon provide much more information. Even today, the work of Falk and Kotin has, to some extent explained why, in spite of the omnipresence of benzpyrene in the human environment, fewer people suffer from cancer than might actually be expected. In the same environment, hidden chemical antagonists constantly thwart the attacks of their carcinogenic rivals.

In the Ben-May Research Institute of Professor Charles Huggins, which began the hormone treatment of cancer of the breast and prostate, mice were protected against hydrocarbons that are normally carcinogenic. From this Huggins drew, in a lecture at Heidelberg in 1965, an extremely optimistic conclusion. "The day is not far off when we shall have powerful compounds with which to immunise our children against chemical carcinogens."

Unfortunately it is doubtful whether this bold prophecy will soon be fulfilled. Although the idea of anticarcinogens is so attractive, there is at present no clue as to how children might be permanently immunised against the continuous effect of carcinogens.

Tomorrow's field of research

However, even before vaccines, "immunity boosters" and anticarcinogens introduce a new era in the campaign against cancer, it should be possible, in the opinion of the World Health Organisation, to avoid about 70 per cent of all cancer diseases by means of suitable preventive measures. The President of the American Cancer Society, Dr. Wendell Scott, says, "we should concentrate all our energies at present on the field of cancer prevention".

Professor Karl Heinrich Bauer, too, untiringly advocates cancer prevention. "The prevention of cancer," he wrote "which many scientists yesterday considered a fantasy, will tomorrow be one of the chief concerns in the campaign against cancer."

Bauer gave three reasons why this branch of research must be given much more attention. At present 48 per cent of all cancer diseases in the favourable Stage I and 67 per cent of those in Stage II remain uncured despite numerous temporary successes.

The Heidelberg scientist finds his second reason in the fact that "cancer increases despite all measures adopted to control it, at least in the annual percentage of fatal cases. This, in an age of implicit belief in progress, is a bitter comment, but it never pays to give a truth a wide berth merely because it is disagreeable."

Finally, Bauer warns of the carcinogenic poisons which accumulate to a disquieting degree in man's industrial environment. Their elimination may be the most important task of all for cancer prophylaxis.

Every cancer has its precancerous stage

One of the greatest Russian authorities on cancer, Professor L. A. Shabad, energetically advocated an extension of preventive measures. "The prevention of cancer," he said "is possible – that is the first and most important conclusion from all our modern knowledge of tumours. An enormous number of experimental investigations with many carcinogenic substances have enabled us to trace the development of tumours stage by stage, and to provide a basis for the prevention of cancer."

According to Shabad, it has been proved without doubt that certain chemical compounds can cause tumours in man. If compounds of this kind were removed from the environment, many cancer diseases could be prevented or considerably reduced. Tumours do not, the Soviet pathologist thinks, appear suddenly, but only after a considerable lapse of time, as the last link in a long chain of pretumourous or precancerous events. "Every cancer," he emphasizes, "has its precancerous stage."

The Soviet investigator distinguishes four different stages in the development of malignant tumours:

1. Diffuse, irregular hyperplasia;
2. Nodular growths;
3. Relatively benign tumours;
4. Malignant tumours.

Thus the precancerous phenomena may be very variable. Inflammatory processes, although they are not in themselves precancerous, may play a part. But they may also be absent. The Soviet cancer investigator sees two ways of overcoming the origination of tumours:

1. By preventing the development of a malignant process. This

could be achieved by the discovery and treatment of precancerous stages in time.

2. By removing the carcinogenic factors from the environment of man.

The more precancerous conditions are investigated, the greater, so Shabad hopes, will be the increase in knowledge of cell changes and pathological processes. Such increased knowledge, combined with increasingly refined methods of investigation, will also lead in future to the earlier discovery of precancerous states. The studies of prophylactic measures which have been customary for a long time in the Soviet Union should help here.

In these ways, thousands of early cases of cancer and hundreds of thousands of precancerous stages have been discovered. The result, in the Soviet Union, has been that the proportion of advanced cases of cancer has fallen from a total of 42 per cent in 1947 to 21.3 per cent in 1960. The percentage of early diagnoses rose correspondingly from 44 per cent in 1949 to 67.7 per cent in 1960.

The number of successfully-treated cancer cases without relapses or metastases increased from 45.8 per cent in 1949 to 76.8 per cent in 1960. In this statement of results, which is without doubt highly impressive, Shabad sees proof that the timely discovery and treatment of precancerous stages would effectively keep the disease within the limits of control. "Adequate treatment of the precancerous condition is a method of preventing cancer."

Tar is cleansed

For the Soviet oncologists, just as for their colleagues in the West, the second and still more important method of cancer prevention lies in cleansing the environment of man from carcinogenic substances. The enormous development of modern industry steadily produces new chemical compounds which must be carefully tested for their possible carcinogenic potency.

In the past man had to restrict himself in this connection to reducing to a minimum, or completely excluding contact with, such compounds by means of technical precautions. Nowadays a considerably more effective advance is possible by means of "decancerisation". Thus the Soviet investigator P. A. Bogorski has proposed an industrial method by which the carcinogenic hydrocarbons, including benzpyrene, are extracted from tar during its distillation to coke. 68 per cent of mice treated with the original tar developed tumours. But the tar from which the carcinogens had been removed caused cancer in only 3.7 per cent of the mice. There is no doubt that there is in this a promising clue to the effective prevention of cancer.

In the Western World also, work is constantly being done to extend the early diagnosis of malignant diseases and to familiarise the population with the chief symptoms. Similarly, precancerous stages, such as chronic gastric ulcers and scars resulting from burns, are given closer attention. Here also, in a "scientific hunt – the – criminal", a search is made for external factors which have proved to be carcinogenic in the human environment or are suspected to be so. The greater our knowledge of this becomes, the sooner can preventive measures be taken and the more promising will they be.

Prevention at its most effective

Naturally, the forms of cancer which are due to external causes offer the best chances of rapid prevention. Such exogenous factors include all the carcinogens and carcinogenic substances in man's environment, whether they have already been identified or not. But the closest attention should be given also to hormonal disturbances, the results of deficiences in the diet and metabolic defects, which influence the occurrence or course of cancer. Among the kinds of cancer which depend directly or indirectly on external factors are many tumours of the respiratory system and of the stomach, intestine and urinary system, of the skin and the mouth, of the organs dependent on hormones, such as the breast, the thyroid and the uterus, and also of the blood and lymphatic systems. About threequarters of all cancerous diseases arise in these organs. Because there are long latent periods, usually lasting years or decades, in the development of almost all the tumours, there are many possibilities of interrupting the carcinogenic process or of stopping it. According to Dr. Scott, of the American Cancer Society, at least three ways of doing this are possible:

1. To prevent altogether the origin of a carcinogenic process.
2. To prevent the development of a tumour:
3. To guard against the continued growth of a tumour by suitable diagnostic methods.

In every case it is better, Scott thinks, to make it impossible for cancer to arise than to treat a tumour that is already established. Therefore all available forces must be devoted to the prevention of cancer, just as they have hitherto been concentrated on its treatment.

Epidemiologists provide many leads towards a possible prevention of cancer. They record indefatigably which kinds of cancer most frequently met in specific parts of the world, and what causes could possibly be concerned in them. Whoever devotes himself to the study of these voluminous reports will, without doubt, encounter many highly contradictory facts. There are, however, many signs that strengthen the suspicion that the origin of cancer is decisively affected by habits of life and environmental factors. The American investigator Earnest Wynder, who has devoted himself completely to the thesis of the external causation of cancer, sees here the most important explanation why the risk of cancer increases with age. Wynder notes two circumstances: the older a person becomes, the greater is the sum of carcinogens to which he has been exposed. Secondly, with advancing age there is a general weakening of the resistant forces of the cells.

Cancer of the mouth in China and Scandinavia

Apart from assessing the age at which cancer attacks man, epidemiologists have tried to prove a striking "preference" in cancers for certain geographical regions. But only rarely is it possible to explain these differences. Thus, for example, in China and some other Asiatic countries, cancer of the mouth, nose and pharynx is especially common. A reason for this could be, experts think, that much betel nut is chewed in these regions. There is also the custom, prevalent in many parts of Asia, of putting the burning ends of cigars into the mouth! But this would be at most only a partial explanation. In Scandinavia, where that strange custom is unknown, the same kinds of cancer have just as often been reported. Available statistical material can give only an inadequate explanation, determined by the limited data that can be obtained. Nevertheless, the World Health Organisation is eager to collect all possible data on the areas that are afflicted particularly often, or particularly seldom, by the various kinds of cancer.

It is clear that cancer of the mouth and pharynx is widely distributed in Ireland, Switzerland and England, but is less often met with in Colombia, Venezuela, Israel and Japan. The incidence of cancer of the cervix is high in Portugal, England, Scotland and Switzerland, but low in Ireland, Japan, Italy and Israel. Cancer of the uterus again is common in Japan, the Federal Republic of Germany, Austria, Belgium and France in comparison with Israel, Norway, Portugal, New Zealand and Holland. Cancer of the bladder is common in England, rare in Japan; cancer of the thyroid is common in Austria and Switzerland, rarer in Germany, Belgium, France, Holland and Australia. The number of leukaemic diseases is highest in the U.S.A., Denmark and Sweden and lowest in Colombia and Ceylon.

Dr. Walter B. Quisenberry carried out similar statistical researches in Hawaii. These were not concerned with geographical differences, but with the frequency of cancer in the various nations and races which meet in Hawaii. The inhabitants there are of Japanese, European, Hawaiian, Philippino and Chinese ancestry, with a smaller percentage of Samoans, Koreans and Puerto Ricans.

Dr. Quisenberry found typical differences in the frequency of individual kinds of cancer, but the search for the causes of these differences were based upon fairly vague suppositions.

Japanese in Hawaii are especially threatened by cancer of the stomach; this way perhaps be traceable to the lower social status of the Japanese population there, and also to the Japanese feeding habits. Cancer of the liver finds its victims especially among the Philipinos, whose diet contains little vitamin B_1, but much carbohydrate. Cancer of the lung is less common in Japanese and Philippino men, most of whom are non-smokers. Cancer of the breast is five times less common among Japanese women than among the women of the other nations; this might relate to the fact that more Japanese women suckle their own children. Cancer of the prostate is found nine times more often among the descendants of European peoples than among the Japanese. Cancer of the pharynx and nose is found among the Chinese, who are accustomed to drinking extremely hot tea.

But all these indications are only vague aids when an explanation is sought as to why the incidence of this or that kind of cancer varies so widely between different regions. Sometimes no suggestions are possible. Thus in Sumatra Chinese workers suffer much more often from cancer of the stomach than do their

Javanese colleagues although they live under the same conditions and eat the same rice food.

Epidemiologists are working intensively all over the world on the contradictory behaviour of cancer of the stomach, which still accounts for the majority of cancer patients. In the United States, carcinoma of the stomach has been in retreat for more than 20 years, during which research indicates a decline of around 50 per cent. On the other hand its incidence is still very high in Japan and Iceland and is increasing in Russia. In Germany it has for some years declined.

Divided opinions on diet

There are whole libraries of scientific literature on a possible relationship between cancer of the stomach and nutrition, and bitter feuds have been fought over the years among scientists. Although it was constantly asserted that cancer, and especially cancer of the stomach, may be avoided by a suitable diet, nothing decisive could be said about this.

Whilst, for example, the Soviet research worker Pokrowski gave his views on possible dietary prevention of cancer to the 7th International Nutritional Congress in Hamburg, Professor Joachim Kühnau advocated the opposite opinion. He is convinced that a large number of the diseases of civilisation can be prevented by correct nutrition, "But unfortunately not the occurrence of cancer!"

The Japanese doctor Takashi Hirayama, however, referred at the IXth International Cancer Research Congress in Tokyo in October, 1966, to statistics indicating that people who drink plenty of milk are threatened less by cancer. The slow decline of cancer of the stomach in Japan might therefore be related to an increase in the consumption of milk. Dr. Hirayama reported, on the other hand, that his own observations on cancer of the stomach implied a positive link with salted foods.

In their search for carcinogenic substances in food, research workers have in the past concentrated especially on smoked meat, smoked fish and grilled steaks, but without decisive results.

Nowadays, on the other hand, more attention is paid to diets very rich in carbohydrate. Cancer of the stomach is prevalent in countries where rice, potatoes and bread are prominent on the menu card. But it is strikingly infrequent where fresh fruit and vegetables are plentifully eaten. Even so, the way in which food is taken seems also to have a certain importance; foods that are too cold or too hot can at least favour the development of cancer of the stomach. Perhaps the present contradictory picture of cancer of the stomach will soon become clearer if research like that begun recently in the Federal Republic of Germany by the Hamburg chemist Dr. Gernot Grimmer are one day applied to the different regions of the world.

Benzpyrene in foods

Grimmer and his colleagues have been concerned with the benzpyrene content of various basic foods, and have obtained results which are as interesting as they are depressing. In order to calculate to 1/10th of a milligram of hydrocarbons in various foods, Grimmer and his colleagues had to devise new and extensive analytical procedures in order to achieve quantitatively accurate results. The result was quite sensational. Grimmer and his team found that vegetables and salads were particularly highly contaminated with hydrocarbons of various kinds. Among them in every instance was the carcinogenic benzpyrene. The highest amount, about 12–24 microgrammes per kilogramme, was found in kale.

Even washed kale still contained 15.6 microgrammes per kilogramme, whilst the water used for washing subsequently showed about 1.0–1.6 microgrammes of 3, 4-benzpyrene. In salads, the benzpyrene content varied between 2.85 microgrammes and 12.8; in spinach it was 7.4, in leeks 6.6 microgrammes.

In order to demonstrate the carcinogenic activity of even such minimal quantities, 80–100 microgrammes (present in about 4 kilogrammes of kale) were enough, when they were injected subcutaneously, to cause tumours in 50 per cent of a colony of mice.

In the same way Grimmer examined cereals, bread, coffee, tea, roasted meat, smoked meats, milk and better.

With cereals 23 tests gave values of between 0.2 and 4.1 microgrammes of benzpyrene, and even flour and bread contained some.

The vindication of smoked meats

"Surprisingly," said Grimmer, "the eleven samples of coffee showed no noteworthy quantities of hydrocarbons." Still, in an aqueous extract of tea, about 4 microgrammes of 3, 4-benzpyrene were found in two tests.

There was an unexpected "vindication" of foods which are subject to the greatest suspicion of carcinogenic properties. Thus Grimmer found that roasted and grilled meats contained hardly any benzpyrene. Also, according to him, smoked meats have only a small content of benzpyrene. Smoked fish contained 0.1–0.8 microgrammes, and sausage cooked in its skin 0.2 microgrammes. Even in the skin of heavily smoked sausage there were only 0.4 microgrammes, whilst the sausage itself contained none. In milk, either in bottles or in paper bags impregnated with paraffin, and in German or Danish market butter, the Hamburg research team found no demonstrable quantities of hydrocarbons.

Presumably the hydrocarbons get into the foodstuffs through the dust and soot in the air. This seems to be supported by analyses of cereals made in various localities. Samples from the Ruhr region contained about 10 times more hydrocarbons than those from Lower Saxony, Holstein or other more rural areas of the Federal Republic of Germany.

The marked fall in cancer of the stomach in the U.S.A. indicates, thinks Dr. Frank Horsfall of the Sloan-Kettering Institute, that hereditary influences must play a smaller part in this kind of cancer than do the effects of the environment. On the other hand, the most recent studies have shown a certain relationship between cancer of the stomach and people who have the genetically determined blood group A. Malignant diseases of the salivary glands are also more common in people with this blood group. Clearly, people with this blood group may show a somewhat higher sensitivity to these two forms of cancer.

However, no grounds can yet be found for these statistical statements, or for the belief that nutritional factors may also play a part in cancer of the intestine.

Nuns and Jewish women are excepted

Statistics, especially those compiled in the United States on genital cancer, can show striking features. They indicate, for example, that cancer of the cervix is extremely rare in Jewish women both in Israel and in other countries of the world. In non-Jewish women, on the other hand, this cancer is 9 times more common. Cancer of the penis, too, is as good as unknown in the Jewish population of New York.

There is at present no scientific explanation of these astonishing facts. However, the implication is that in both cases hygiene plays a great part. Indications of this are given by investigations which show that there are apparently carcinogenic substances in the smegma which collects under the male foreskin though experiments on animals reported to the German Cancer Congress in Münich this year by Dr. Matthias Krahe showed that the smegma itself is clearly not carcinogenic.

American statistics point in the same direction: cancer of the cervix is an extremely rare event in Catholic nuns. These tumours are especially common in the American Negro population. There was, in the white population of America between 1930 and 1960, a decrease of 50 per cent of cancer of the cervix, but in the Negro population the decrease was only 25 per cent.

Professor Ernest L. Wynder of the New York Sloan-Kettering Institute for Cancer Research therefore stressed the importance of strict hygiene. This is important enough in man, because carcinoma of the penis is practically never found in circumcised men, but it is still more important in women. Probably the epithelium of the portio in women is more liable to cancer than the male epithelium is. "I think," Professor Wynder emphasized, "that this is a very important point in the prevention of cancer."

Interesting material on this question came from Professor William M. Christopherson of the Medical Faculty of the University of Louisville, Kentucky. According to him, women who have married at the age of 19 or earlier suffer especially often from cancer of the uterus. Strong sexual activity, especially if it begins at a relatively early age, increases, the risk of cancer of the uterus, Christopherson deduced. The fact that this form of cancer may be so common in the American Negro population is due rather to this than to racial factors. The black population marry on an average one year earlier, and the first pregnancy occurs 3 years earlier than it does among white American women.

Other statistical results must also be mentioned in relation to cancer of the uterus, which, Wynder thinks, depends very much on body weight. It particularly attacks women who are overweight. Possibly an explanation of this is that, when weight is excessive, there are more steroids present in the body.

On the other hand the contraceptive pills used nowadays by millions of women seems to have no carcinogenic effect. Prominent American scientists even believe, after years of investigation, that their effect may be to prevent cancer.

Only two per cent of errors

It cannot be emphasized often enough that carcinoma of the cervix offers the best prospects of cure if it is treated early. In such cases the chance of recovery is 98 per cent. Relapses or metastases are practically unknown.

But in cancer of the cervix it is not only therapeutic successes that give cause for hope. As has already been described in Chapter 2, there is also a method of early detection which is as simple as it is sure, which makes possible the certain diagnosis of cancer before it has become dangerous: the smear. In cervical cancer, the cells of the mucosa on the surface are affected in the preliminary stage of the disease. When smears of them are examined by experts, there is at present an error of only 2 per cent. Centres which use this diagnostic method have for some years existed in all the Universities and in many large hospitals in the Federal Republic of Germany. Their work is very successful. Unfortunately many women are not fully aware that an incomparable opportunity is in this way offered to them to avoid one of the greatest threats to health. If they would undergo an annual cytological examination, cancer of the cervix would probably lose all its terrors.

The example of New York State showed this most convincingly. Here, all the women more than 35 years old are obliged by law to allow themselves to be examined once a year. The result in the State of New York is that cancer of the cervix has been almost eliminated.

In the Federal Republic of Germany however, legal measures of a similar kind would be premature, because there are still too few medical experts and technical personnel to organise as many centres of investigation as would be necessary. But certainly this would be different if enough women recognised the prospects for a genuine prophylaxis.

Shocks in the Terry report

Although cancer investigators are not fully agreed about the part played by environmental influences, their opinion is, in one respect, almost unanimous: there is a direct relationship between smoking and lung cancer. The most comprehensive report on this subject was published in 1964 in the United States, and became known through the headlines of the world press as "The Terry Report". In it, all the research hitherto carried out was stringently evaluated and summarised in an impressive general view.

The most shocking fact presented was that, whilst in the year 1930 fewer than 3,000 cases of death from lung cancer were recorded, this number rose to more than 41,000 in 1962.

Experiments on animals showed that at least seven chemical compounds, present in tobacco smoke or tar products, cause cancer if they are applied to the skin of mice or rabbits or are injected subcutaneously into rats.

Because the results of experiments on animals cannot be directly applied to the effects on man, these observations would in themselves not signify too much. They attained their full threatening character only in the light of statistical investigations, in which the health of more than a million Americans was observed for many years. The results of these studies speak for themselves.

Cigarettes are the most dangerous

The total death rate among smokers was 68 per cent higher than among non-smokers. This number includes all causes of death. But in lung cancer the result was still more startling. The mortality among smokers was almost 1,000 per cent higher than that among non-smokers. Among smokers the mortality due to some other forms of cancer was also considerably higher: up to 440 per cent in cancer of the air passages, up to 310 per cent in cancer of the mouth, up to 240 per cent in cancer of the oesophagus, up to 90 per cent in cancer of the bladder and 50 per cent in cancer of the kidneys.

The investigations further showed the smoker to be increasingly endangered by the number of cigarettes he smokes each day, the age at which he begins to smoke and the degree to which he inhales.

The risk among cigar and pipe smokers is much smaller than it is among cigarette smokers. This seems chiefly attributable to the fact the cigar-smokers and pipe smokers inhale much less. However, among pipe smokers the incidence of cancer of the lips is above the average.

Obviously every cancer of the lung is not due to smoking, and even when its cause is an excessive consumption of cigarettes, other factors may often co-operate. The pollution of the air in industrial centres, and that caused by traffic, certainly plays a strong, and possibly dominant part in lung cancer. Professor Otto Hettche the Essen hygienist presented very interesting figures on this subject to the 1965 Congress in Medical Continuation Studies in Berlin. According to these, inhabitants of large towns inhale, in a year, about 280 gamma of benzpyrene. One gamma corresponds to one thousandth of a milligramme.

If one considers that 50 cigarettes contain about one gamma of this carcinogen, it is not difficult to calculate that the inhabitant of a large town pumps into his lungs every day the benzpyrene equivalent of 40 cigarettes.

English studies also attach special importance to air pollution as a source of lung cancer. According to these, a non-smoker in an English industrial city like Liverpool, breathes in an amount of benzpyrene about 14 times greater than does a smoker in the pure air of the Alps. In Germany, too, there is an obvious relationship between lung cancer and the density of the population and of industry.

The disastrous contribution made by car exhaust gases has not yet been sufficiently investigated. But it can hardly be denied any longer that motorists who battle daily through air polluted by exhaust gases in large towns, are exposed far more to the risk of bronchial carcinoma than are travellers in rural areas.

The most recently published measurements of the benzpyrene content of automobile exhaust gases emphasize this risk most emphatically. According to these, a heavy lorry, parked for a few minutes with its engine running, produces as much of this carcinogen as an average cigarette smoker does in more than 20 years. A lorry with a higher oil consumption – especially the type that uses a mixture of oil and benzine – which travels for a bare 3 hours in a large town of, say, 600,000 inhabitants, produces the same amount of benzpyrene as the whole population do with their cigarettes.

Certainly, in the future, many more investigations will be done on the various causes of lung cancer. The cigarette will then be found only partially to blame. Nevertheless, it is surprising that many investigators refuse to consider smoking to be at least one of the two dominating factors. Among them for example, is Professor Heinz Oeser, Director of the X-ray Clinic in the Free University of Berlin.

In spite of the impressive statistics, Oeser holds the opinion that smoking does not encourage lung cancer. In a letter to the author Oeser wrote: "We should not, in the search for the cause of cancer, allow ourselves to be governed by a single idea, as happened in the crusades of the Middle Ages." The relationships of carcinogenesis may be much more complex. "One cannot speak of a close causal relationship between smoking and carcinoma of the lung."

Naturally Oeser does not in any way deny the increase of lung cancer. But, he emphasizes, a decline of other forms of cancer contrast with it – for example, of cancer of the stomach may remain unchanged. From this it can be conluded that environmental factors have had no influence on the total incidence of cancer. Professor Oeser's colleague, K. Rach, even quotes statistics which indicate that in Germany, since 1935, progressively fewer women than men died of cancer of the respiratory organs, although more and more women smoke. In 1935 this relationship was 100:37, but in 1961 only 100:17.

More than respiration is endangered

Oeser, however, finds himself in "splendid isolation" in his opinion. Most other experts are thoroughly convinced that a definite relationship is evident between smoking and the steeply rising number of lung cancer cases. Moreover, the suspicion has increased that the use of tobacco does not cause lung cancer alone. Smoking seems, though to a smaller degree, to encourage cancer of the bladder.

The Terry Report gave statistical evidence of this. However, statistics alone do not represent scientific proof. It is not possible fully to explain the data they offer. Still, a relationship between smoking and lung cancer is quite easy to understand. When cigarette smoke is inhaled, the bronchi come directly and constantly into contact with the tarry substances in the smoke. But, if cigarettes are responsible for the increasing incidence of cancer of the bladder, other mechanisms, at present unknown, must be operative.

Recent research carried out by Dr. William Kerr of the Banting Institute of the University of Toronto, Canada, seem to represent a tiny step forward. Kerr started with experiments on mice. If the bladders of these animals was brought into contact with chemical compounds from human urine, cancer could be caused in them. These chemicals were certain ortho-amino phenol compounds, metabolic products of tryptophane. Remarkably large quantities of them were also found in the excretions of patients suffering from cancer of the bladder.

Kerr investigated a group of six people composed of smokers and non-smokers. The urine of the smokers was analysed several times, at the time when they smoked and also during periods of 3 weeks to 3 months during which they temporarily abstained. The same experiment was done with the non-smokers, who declared themselves ready to smoke for a period of 3 weeks.

The experiments showed without exception that cigarette smoking considerably increased the amount of carcinogenic ortho-amino phenol in the urine. There was an average increase of 37 per cent, but in individual cases it was as high as 64 per cent. During the period when there was no smoking the proportion of the carcinogen decreased.

Kerr therefore supposed that smoking impeded or inhibited the normal decomposition of tryptophane and for this reason more of the carcinogenic metabolites of tryptophane accumulated in the urine. Because these products remained for a long time in the urinary system, carcinoma of the bladder could ultimately arise ."This opens up a completely new field of cancer research," commented Dr. Clifford Ashe, Director of the Ontario Cancer Institute.

A number of authors, among them Dr. Hans Ehrhart of the Munich University Medical Clinic had earlier noted the fact that metabolic products of tryptophane cause leukaemia in mice.

Antibiotics as diagnostic agents

The diagnosis of cancer of the bladder, like the detection of early metastases in bones, may be improved considerably in the future. At least, extensive research work recently carried out in the Sloan-Kettering Institute suggests this. Blood in the urine, malignant cells in smears from the urethra, inspection of the bladder by means of the cystoscope and even the removal of minute pieces of tissue, cannot always provide definite evidence of this disease. In particular, they cannot provide accurate information about the site of the tumour.

However, since it has been found in the Sloan-Kettering Institute that the frequently-used antibiotic tetracycline concentrates preferentially in tumours of the bladder and shows fluorescence under ultraviolet light, there is hope of much earlier diagnosis in the future. The extent to which this excellent method can also be used for cancer of the lungs or stomach is being at present studied. Contrasted with these investigations are a series of experiments in which Dr. Gericke and his colleagues of Farbwerke Hoechst found that tetracycline had no specific affinity for solid tumour tissue.

1,400 doctors consider prevention

What possibilities of preventing cancer are seen by doctors who deal almost daily with cases of the disease in all its stages and who, between them, have thousands of case histories? An attempt to obtain answers to this question was made by an enquiry organised in 1957–1961 by Dr. Robert J. Samp of the University of Wisconsin, on behalf of the American Cancer Society. No fewer than 1,400 doctors in the State were interviewed by letter. By far the majority of them were agreed on one point – that excessive irradiation with X-rays or excessive influences of radioactive substances should be avoided in all circumstances. This should be measure No. 1 in the prophylaxis of cancer.

Many doctors also considered that prompt therapeutic or surgical treatment is necessary in a number of complaints. Unfortunately, symptoms of these are too often ignored. Yet they might possibly be identified as precursors of cancer. Thus polyps in the intestine or bladder, large cysts and growths in the ovary, and nodules in the thyroid gland should be removed and their tissue examined under the microscope for malignant cells. All chronic infections of the cervix should be carefully treated. In addition it was recommended that Pap-smears should be done on all adult women in order to detect possibly abnormal cells in the uterus. These measures were advocated by between 700 and 1,000 doctors.

The views expressed on other preventive measures were not so clear, and less than half of the doctors mentioned them. They included surgical investigation of suspected growths in the female breast or warts on the skin, and the prompt treatment of gastric ulcers, chronic gastritis, pernicious anaemia, chronic throat infections and dental troubles.

The doctors were unanimous about the advisability of the circumcision in male babies. They stressed that the population must be better protected from the common carcinogens in the dust from asphalted and tarred streets, in exhaust gases and food-additives. They warned against the uncontrolled use of chemotherapeutic substances, especially hormone and arsenical preparations. Tobacco, they insisted, should be avoided in all its forms. The skin should not come into contact with tar and petroleum products.

Comparatively few of the doctors considered it risky to take very hot foods, drinks, large quantities of alcohol, or excessively strong spices, or to use purgatives.

What conclusions can be drawn?

Naturally, a compendium of preventive measures against cancer can never at present be complete. It is certain that by no means all the carcinogenic substances in the human environment have yet been discovered and that much further research is needed to explain more clearly the effect of substances so far suspected of being carcinogenic. But it is important that conclusions should be drawn by doctors, the general public, and the State authorities, from the scientific results so far obtained.

Although it may sound strange to many ears, much must be done to inform doctors themselves before the prevention of cancer can be developed on a broad front. It is precisely from them that the most uncomfortable questions come! What is the use of pointing out to the public the early symptoms of cancer, and persuading more and more people to seek routine annual examinations if many doctors are not sufficiently versed in the modern methods of investigation?

Statistics cannot record the consequences of a negligent attitude nor can they show how often the most favourable time for the treatment of definite tumours is missed nor how often as a result a definitely curable cancer becomes incurable. But a considerable number of cancer case histories reveal an inexcusable disregard of the early symptoms by the doctor who first treated them.

The annual medical examinations which, in the opinion of the American Cancer Society, are so important for people over 35, should not only include thorough physical examination from head to toe, but also the most modern radiological checks, and tests of the blood and other body fluids. The intestinal region should be examined both manually and with the aid of endoscopes.

But clinical methods, too, must be greatly improved in many kinds of cancer. Although medical ability and experience has increased so much in the large universities, about 25–30 per cent of all cancerous diseases still remain undetected. "That means that only about 75 per cent of all cancers are diagnosed before death. The remainder first come to light at the post mortem stage, as a discovery which no doctor suspected." This sentence came from the well-known specialist Dr. Siegfried Heyden in Switzerland.

According to Heyden's report the percentage of undiagnosed cancers is highest in organs which are not normally attacked by cancer – the kidneys, liver, testes and gall bladder. Only when new diagnostic methods are successfully developed can this alarmingly high percentage of undiagnosed cancers be reduced to any degree.

"The only possibility of abolishing the terrors of this disease," said Professor Graffi, in Berlin-Buch, "lies in constant study of precautions. We must pursue this line, which can help to solve the cancer problem by at least 50 per cent.

"These studies however," confirmed Graffi, "involve considerable expenditure." The annual budget of his East Berlin Institute amounts at present to about £600,000. It has some 50 scientific workers, of whom 30 work in the clinical division of the Robert-Roessle Clinic; the other 20 are occupied with experimental cancer research in the Institute, which is part of a medical and biological research organisation with a total of eight research centres.

According to Graffi, research establishments alone achieve nothing. In his opinion the development of diagnosis by means of modern instruments, such as those used for the inspection of the intestine and stomach, is just as important. "This naturally requires considerable finance, but it would permit the early diagnosis and treatment of at least three quarters of all cases of cancer."

Graffi also considers it an advantage that in the DDR cancer is a notifiable disease, and this provides his Institute with complete statistics from which valuable conclusions can be drawn.

"Moreover it also helpful to prophylaxis that all cigarette advertising is forbidden in our country."

However, even if one day the disease should have been reduced to second place among the causes of death, human research activity will still not be content. It will not rest until the reason why cells become malignant has been explained, and it is known what processes and reactions in the body play a part in this.

Nobody can predict how long these struggles between man and disease will last. The immense cost of cancer research in many countries of the world has been reported in detail in the preceding chapters. Progress is clearly dependent upon results in the spheres of biology, embryology, genetics, and many other disciplines. And there is still the possibility that one of the decisive discoveries will be made by a scientist who is not working in cancer research at all.

Review of the major hypotheses

Perhaps it may be found that so many of the ideas and hypotheses with which science has previously tried to explain the phenomena of malignant cells, contained at least a grain of truth and were partially adequate to explain some of the phenomena of cancer.

In this book it has been possible to give only a review of the most important hypotheses: Virchow's irritation theory, according to which in cells exposed to constant external stimuli the hereditary substance is altered and they become malignant. Or Julius Cohnheim's embryonal theory, which postulates that "unused" embryonal cells persist after the developmental stage of the organism, and years later begin suddenly to multiply uncontrollably and unrestrainedly.

The new century then brought plenty of additional ideas about the mysterious processes which convert a healthy cell into a malignant one. The most popular of these was the mutation theory of Karl Heinrich Bauer.

A change in the hereditary substance of the cell, whether it were spontaneous or due to chemicals or radiation, could be the cause of the birth of anew and malignant strain of cells. This idea was developed by other research workers: who thought that cancer need not arise entirely from a mutation in the genes in the cell nucleus, but might be, under certain conditions, traced to changes in the plasma genes.

As more knowledge was gained about the nucleic acids, especially about DNA, the more closely did it become connected with the mutation theory. And the basic concept of the theory remained unaffected by this.

The German Nobel Prize Laureate Otto Warburg categorically declared enphatically that a conversion of the metabolism of the cell from respiration to fermentation may be the real evil, whilst other scientists thought that disturbances in the hormone economy were responsible for the formation of cancerous tumours.

These ideas were finally supplemented by the immunological theory especially advocated by Professor Green in Leeds. According to this, the cancer cell has lost tissue specific antigens and can therefore no longer be prevented by the surrounding tissue from undergoing irregular and unrestrained growth.

The virus theory also gains in popularity. According to this, viruses play a definite part, at least in some forms of cancer in animals.

The opposition dwindles

For some decades, two theories were particularly opposed to each other as rivals. One saw cancer as the result of a mutation in the body cells, the other attributed the reponsibility to viruses. Nowadays comparatively few scientists believe the opposition of these theories to be irreconcilable. Since the molecular approach has gained ground and viruses are now regarded as being migratory genemolecules.

According to this expanded theory, viruses, with their DNA or RNA complex, are ultimately nothing but mutagenic factors. They act much more directly on the nucleic acids of a host cell than do chemical substances, and upset the mechanism of heredity and control.

"At the very beginning it is a question of an intracellular phenomenon of body cells, in which a change (mutation) is brought about by injuries inflicted from the outside on the submicroscopic genetic basis of cell division (and through this of tissue growth). Such a process is not reversible, but on the other hand transmits its effect according to a new code to all the subsequent descendants of the cell. Their growth, in contrast to that of the body cells, becomes autonomous. Cancer cells are subject to a new order to behave themselves as they must do, even in cancer."

These sentences written by Professor Bauer, are taken from an article in the "Frankfürter Allgemeinen Zeitung" which appeared in October 1964, on the occasion of the inauguration of the first section of the German cancer research centre in Heidelberg.

And whether Professor Bauer himself is unwilling to believe so much in the virus etiology of human cancer also, it can easily be reconciled with his conception of mutation in the body cells. Among the "injuries from the outside" which act on the hereditary substance of these body cells viruses must be included, together with chemical substances and irradiation. This has been decisively proved by thousands of experiments on animals.

Whilst the mutation theory – though it is presented so attractively – is at present not experimentally demonstrable in any form, virus etiology has a solid foundation in experiments on animals. Because nobody can today deny that many animal tumours are definitely caused by viruses, it is very difficult to conceive that viruses should be oncogenic only in animals and not in man. "It becomes more and more improbable," said the American Nobel Laureate John Enders, "that man should be excepted from a phenomenon which can be so readily and so often caused in a whole series of species."

And one of the most reowned German virologists Professor Werner Schäfer, of the Max-Planck Institute for virus investigation, in his ceremonial lecture in the Therapy Week at Karlsruhe in 1966, expressed himself in a similar way: "As a virologist I must here express the conviction that viruses are not at all the only causes of malignant tumours in man, but are only one of these causes."

And in another place: "Plainly in our country the occurrence of viruses that cause tumours in man is always disputed, although meanwhile it has been definitely proved that viruses can cause tumours in the most different kinds of animals up to the monkeys. I don't see why man should differ in just this respect from the other mammals including the primates."

But meanwhile the virologists are also unable to make any reply. They play, as has been already mentioned, the part of public prosecutor who has collected an almost unbroken chain of evidence with painstaking care. However, the last link which would definitely convict the culprits, is still lacking.

However, even if this final proof should one day be achieved, it is certain that only some cancers are caused by viruses. And it cannot be said with certainty whether cancer always comes from without, whether it is acquired and therefore must be ascribed to exogenous agencies or whether many kinds of cancer have purely endogenous causes.

Possibly the causal chain of cancer is on the whole much longer than has been hitherto supposed. A co-operation of external and internal factors, which the Basle surgeon Professor Rudolf Nissen, for example, assumed to be the prerequisite for cancerous disease, cannot in any way be excluded. In many kinds of cancer it acquires more and more probability. According to Nissen a fateful internal factor is responsible for the disease itself and for the disposition to it. External factors on the other hand such as the effects of radiation, chemical substances or other injuries determine the site at which the tumours are formed.

Many research workers think that many people have a liability to cancer. The pathologist Bernhard Fischer-Wasels, who worked in Frankfurt University in the thirties, considered that an inherited liability to cancer is proved: "For the origin of a tumour, in addition to local factors (embryonic germ, focus of regeneration), the general factor, the total disposition of the body to the formation of a new strain of cells, is necessary." The local factor, like the general factor, can be inherited. But it could also be acquired through typical injuries. It may also be possible that one factor is inherited and the other acquired.

Fischer-Wasels was not disconcerted by the practice of surgery by which removal of tumours led to cure. He replied that the general factor is, in fact, not excluded by the operation, but is doubtless influenced by it. If a tumour should be removed, the organism can subsequently recover so far, "that now the general disposition also subsides or disappears".

However, even today the dispute is unresolved as to whether cancer is initially a purely local disease, or a generalised one which is simply manifested at a certain site. As has already been mentioned, the results of research during recent decades have tipped the balances distinctly in favour of those who regard cancer as a local disease. But, in this sphere also, a final decision will only be possible in the future.

Biochemical knowledge nowadays accumulates to such an

imposing degree that results of research so far done cannot claim any general validity. Cancer constantly enforces exceptions, so that results that are apparently well-established must be continually qualified. Whether it is a question of etiology, pathogenesis or clinical prognosis and treatment, science has nowhere, in spite of the many individual scientific results, reached a point at which statements free from doubt are possible.

H. G. Wells suggested that the riddle of cancer will certainly one day be solved by man. The powerful activating force here may not so much be man's compassion for his fellow creatures, as the irresistible urge to examine creation in its mysterious workshop.

Dr. Michael B. Shimkin, one of the leading American cancer experts often cited in this book, found a comforting picture in his outline of the present position of cancer research. Although, for many laymen, the results so far obtained may not be clearly comprehensible, knowledge of cancer nowadays accumulates, Shimkin thought, on a scale and at a speed as has never before been achieved. The consequence of that may not be immediately evident, but knowledge and insight into the innermost nature of this plague of our age increase like water behind a dam. For the time being this has no consequence; but when the mass of water reaches the uppermost rim of the dam, everything will happen with lightning speed.

Attacks on the molecules of life

Already mankind has learned something of the architectural patterns of the life hidden in the nucleic acids. Already scientists know some of the most important principles, the primary biochemical codes by which DNA dictates the formation of new cells and heredity. As knowledge of this vital compound grows, it becomes increasingly evident that it is in the nucleic acids that thousands of the co-ordinates of cancer research meet – that all roads end, from whatever starting point the scientist approach the cancer problem. Recent results show that there can no longer be any doubt that this is the direction which will lead to ultimate success. Perhaps it will then emerge that cancer, as such, has never actually existed, but that there is rather an interlinked group of separate diseases, which arise from quite different causes – curable by a broad range of biochemical attacks on the molecule of life.

When the great battle for life in thousands of laboratories nears its end, mankind may actually stand on the very threshold of creation, faced not only by the question, what is cancer? but also what is life? Perhaps then it will seem ironical that the disease that has brought death to so many people should have contributed so much to the investigation of the most mysterious mechanisms of life.

BIBLIOGRAPHY

Many of the quotations given in this book are from conversations between the author and the scientist concerned, or from records made available to him. Otherwise, from the many publications used, the following may be regarded as the most important:

Bauer, Karl Heinrich: *Das Krebsproblem.* Springer-Verlag, Berlin 1963.

Berenblum, I.: *Man against Cancer.* The Johns Hopkins Press, Baltimore 1952.

Blohmke, Maria und Schaefer, Hans: *Erfolge und Grenzen der modernen Medizin.* Fischer Bücherei, Frankfurt a. M. 1966.

Clayson, David B.: *Chemical Carcinogenesis.* J. & A. Churchill, Ltd., London 1962.

Considine, Bob: *That Many may live.* Memorial Center for Cancer and Allied Diseases, New York.

Coult, D. A.: *Molecules and Cells.* Longmans, Green & Co. Ltd., London 1966.

Curtis, Helena: *The Viruses.* The Natural History Press, Garden City, New York 1965.

Graffi, Arnold und Bielka, Heinz: *Probleme der experimentellen Krebsforschung.* Akademische Verlagsgesellschaft Geest & Portig, Leipzig 1959.

Harbers, Eberhard, Domagk, Götz F. und Müller, Werner: *Die Nucleinsäuren.* Georg Thieme Verlag, Stuttgart 1964.

McElroy, William D.: *Biochemie und Physiologie der Zelle.* Kosmos Franckh'sche Verlagshandlung, Stuttgart 1964.

McGrady, Pat: *The Savage Cell.* Basic Books, Inc., Publishers, New York 1964.

Meythaler, Friedrich: *Therapie maligner Tumoren, Hämoblastome und Hämoblastosen. I. Band Pathologie und Chemotherapie.* Ferdinand Encke-Verlag, Stuttgart 1966.

Mollowitz, G.: *Kleine Krebsfibel.* Johann Ambrosius Barth, München 1964.

Muller, Hermann Joseph: *Studies in Genetics.* Indiana University Press, Bloomington 1962.

Oberling, Charles: *Krebs, das Rätsel seiner Entstehung.* Rowohlt, Hamburg 1959.

Shimkin, Michael B.: *Science and Cancer.* Public Health Service Publication No. 1162, New York 1964.

Swanson, Carl P.: *Die Zelle.* Kosmos Franckh'sche Verlagshandlung, Stuttgart 1964.

Taylor, Gordon Rattray: *Das Wissen vom Leben.* Droemersche Verlagsanstalt Th. Knaur Nachf., München/Zürich 1963.

Weisburger, John N. und Weisburger, Elisabeth K.: *Chemicals as Causes of Cancer.* Chemical & Engineering News, New York 1966.

The American Cancer Society, Inc.: *Smoking and Health.* New York.

–: *Ca – A Cancer Journal for Clinicans.* New York 1965.

British Empire Cancer Campaign for Research: *Forty-Third Annual Report.* London 1965.

British Medical Bulletin: *Causation of Cancer.* London 1958.

–: *Mechanisms of Carcinogenesis: Chemical, Physical and Viral.* London 1964.

The Imperial Cancer Research Fund: *Sixty-First Annual Report and Accounts.* London 1964.

–: *Sixty-Third Annual Report and Accounts.* London 1966.

Institut National de la Santé et de la Recherche Médicale & Association Claude-Bernard: *Institut de Cancérologie et d'Immunogénétique.*

International Union against Cancer: *Activities Report.* Genf.

Medical World News, Part 2. January 1966.

Memorial Sloan Kettering Cancer Center: *Third Report.* New York 1962 und 1963.

–: *Fourth Report.* New York 1964.

Sloan-Kettering-Institute for Cancer Research: *Progress Report XIII.* New York 1960.

–: *Progress Report XVI, Enzymes and Cancer.* New York 1964.

TECHNICAL TERMS BRIEFLY EXPLAINED

Adenoid, gland-like.

Adeno-viruses, a group of viruses which causes illness related to the common cold in man.

Aerobe, living in the presence of oxygen.

Agar-agar a gelatinous material obtained from algae, which is used, among other things, as a nutrient medium in bacteriology.

Alkylating substances, substances which can transfer the hydrocarbon radical (=alkyl) to sites in organic molecules (such as proteins) which are reactive.

Allergy, hypersensitivity of the body to stimuli produced by certain substances, the allergens. Such allergens are, for example, found in the pollen of grasses, strawberries, primroses, milk, flour, the hairs of animals. Allergy diseases include hay fever, asthma, nettle rash, eczema etc.

Alpha rays, Helium nuclei with two positive charges sent out at high speed by radioactive elements.

Amino acids, organic acids, the building materials of proteins and polypeptides. More than 20 are known. The amino acids and their derivatives are very important for metabolism. Certain amino acids, which are absolutely necessary but which the body cannot synthesize for itself, are called essential amino acids. They must be supplied in the protein of the food.

Anaerobic, living in the absence of oxygen, without oxygen.

Anaemia, poverty of the blood, abnormal reduction of the blood pigment and of the red blood cells. Most anaemias are the consequence of diseases and are therefore called secondary anaemias. Causes can be: copious haemorrhages, continuous minor losses of blood as in ulcers of the stomach and intestine, tumours (gastric cancer), poisonings or faulty nutrition. Pallor, lassitude, and weakness are chief symptoms of anaemia. In severe cases there may be fainting, noises in the ears and palpitations of the heart. Secondary anaemias are differentiated from primary anaemias, which include pernicious anaemia and chlorosis.

Anatomy, the science of the structure of the body and of its parts.

Antibiotics, singular; antibiotic. Drugs belonging to chemotherapeutics, metabolic products of fungi, bacteria, algae etc. Antibiotics can to some extent be made synthetically. They inhabit the growth and attacking power of many causes of disease and are therefore used against infectious diseases. There are antibiotics which are effective only against a few causes of disease and others that are effective against many of them. Among the well-known antibiotics are penicillin, streptomycin, tetracycline etc.

Anticarcinogens, substances that act against the causes of cancer.

Antigens, substances (for example, proteins of a foreign kind, constituents of bacteria and viruses) which cause the formation of antibodies in a living organism.

Antibodies, substances which arise as a specific reaction to antigens. They are protective substances, which can abolish the injurious effects of antigens. They play a great part in immunity.

Antimetabolites, substances which, because of their chemical similarity to metabolites, are able to replace them. But, because they do not take on the work of the metabolites, they prevent important processes in the cell, which can die as a result. On the other hand, it has been possible to produce antimetabolites which influence processes in the cell in such a way as to achieve successes in the campaign against cancer.

Antimitotics, substances which can prevent the division of the cell. Among them are, for example, the alkaloid colchicine, the toxin of meadow saffron.

Asbestosis, a disease due to the constant inhalation of air containing asbestos dust. It occurs in workers employed in the asbestos industry. The fine asbestos dust penetrates into the lung tissue which gradually undergoes a pathological change. Symptoms of the disease are cough, dyspnoea, breathlessness. Asbestosis can develop into lung cancer (asbestos cancer).

Aseptic, free from germs or causes of disease.

Aetiology, the science of the causes of disease.

Atypical, departing from the rule or the average, not typical.

Auto-antibodies, antibodies which act against substances in their own body. Their formation depends on a failure of regulation in the body. See horror autotoxicus, auto-immunity, erythematodes.

Auto-immunity, immunity due to auto-antibodies. It can cause the above diseases.

Autopsy, post-mortem, the opening and dissection of the corpse – usually to discover the cause of death.

Bacteria, singular; bacterium. Small unicellular forms of life. Many, but by no means all of them, are causes of disease. Most of them can be made visible under the light microscope. The bacterium consists of an equivalent of the nucleus and of cell plasma and a cell wall. Some bacteria are enclosed in a capsule or a layer of mucus. Many have flagella – mobile organs – projecting from the cell wall. Bacteria can be cultivated on synthetic fluids free from cells and on solid nutrient media. Among diseases caused by bacteria are tuberculosis, diphtheria, anthrax, tetanus, plague, cholera, and typhus.

Bacteriophages, viruses which specifically attack bacteria and multiply in and destroy them. They are very important for research, especially virus research. They can readily and rapidly multiply in cultures of bacteria.

Bacteriostatic, inhibiting or injuring bacteria.

Bacteriocidal, killing or destroying bacteria.

Basalioma, basal cell cancer, a malignant tumour of the skin, especially of the face. It begins as nodules and grows only slowly.

Benign, non-malignant, not fatal.

Beta-rays, electrons sent out at high speed from radioactive elements. They are used, like gamma rays (q.v.) for the deep treatment of malignant tumours. See betatron.

Betatron, electron gun. An apparatus for obtaining beta-rays or utra short-wave X-rays.

Biochemistry, the science of the chemical composition of living things and the chemical processes in them, for example, respiration, digestion, internal and external secretions.

Biocatalysts, see catalysts.

Biopsy the removal of pieces of tissue or of fluid for investigation and the diagnosis of disease. In excision, a piece of tissue is separated with a knife; in puncture, fluid is removed with a hollow needle. Biopsy is a valuable aid to the diagnosis of cancer.

Blood poverty, see anaemia.

Blood picture, an evaluation of the blood by which the red and the white blood corpuscles are counted and the blood pigment is determined. The colour index (the ratio of the blood pigment to the number of red blood corpuscles) is calculated and a drop of blood is treated with a stain by which the blood corpuscles are coloured differently according to their type, structure and state of health.

Departures from the normal blood picture indicate pathological changes in the body. In infectious diseases, the white blood corpuscles appear in increased numbers, and in anaemia the number of red blood corpuscles is reduced. In anaemia the haemoglobin content is also reduced.

Blood pigment, see Haemoglobin.

Blood corpuscles, Red – see erythrocytes
White – see leucocytes.

Blood plasma, the blood fluid, in which are carried the red and white blood corpuscles, the blood platelets and the fibrin which enables the blood to clot. The blood plasma is composed of 90 per cent of water and 7–8 per cent of proteins. It also contains mineral substances, protein derivatives, fats and carbohydrates, enzymes and all the hormones. It can be preserved and stored (plasma conserve).

Blood plasma expanders, fluids with a high molecular proportion of, for example, dextran or gelatine, which help to bolster the circulation when there has been great loss of blood.

Blood platelets, thrombocytes, formed constituents of the blood which float in the blood plasma. Their site of origin is still disputed. They play an important part in the coagulation of the blood.

Blood Sedimentation, a procedure which depends on the characteristic of the blood corpuscles to settle into layers in still blood which has been rendered uncoagulable. Above the sedimented white and red blood corpuscles the clear blood plasma remains. The blood sedimentation rate can be read off in a graduated glass tube. The normal blood sedimentation rate in the male is up to 9 mm. in the first hour, and in women up to 12 mm. After the second hour in the male it is up to 15 mm. and in the female up to 20 mm. If the rate is increased, a pathological change in the body must be inferred, for example, an infectious disease or even cancer.

Blood serum, the fluid discharged during blood coagulation – the blood plasma without the blood corpuscles, blood platelets and fibrin. It contains, after recovery from a disease or after a protective inoculation, a certain proportion of protective substances (antibodies) acting against causes of disease or their toxins. The protective substances can be taken from animals to which toxins have been arificially administered (inoculations) and can be used in serum treatment.

Bronchoscopy, inspection of the interior of the branches (bronchi) of the trachea by means of a tube (bronchoscope) provided with an illuminating source. Fine instruments, introduced through this tube, can remove external foreign bodies or remove pieces of tissue for investigation.

Cancerogenesis, the origin of cancer.

Carcinogens, substances causing cancer. Some of the most widely known are arsenic, chrome, uranium, radium, aniline derivatives, tar, butter yellow, X-rays, radioactive rays.

Carcinoma, a cancer tumour, especially the malignant tumour of epithelial tissues and of the skin and mucosae.

Catalysts, substances which can accelerate or retard chemical reactions, without being themselves altered. Such a process is called catalysis. Bio-catalysts are enzymes, hormones and vitamins.

Cauterisation, destruction of tissues by agents which burn or are caustic.

Cell, the basic constituent of the living thing, the smallest unit of life. Animal cells contain the cell nucleus, the cell plasma and mitochondria. The cell membrane forms the limiting surface between the cell and its environment. New cells arise by division.

Cervix, neck, especially the neck of the uterus.

Chemotherapeutics, drugs, which act by reason of their chemical composition. They are able to destroy causes of disease in the blood or in organs (bactericides) or to affect them too such an extent (bacteriostatic) that the defensive substances of the body are able to deal with the causes of disease. Among them are sulphonamides, antimalarial drugs, antibiotics, arsenical, bismuth and antimonial preparations. When they are administered they act in the body against infectious causes of disease but not on the body cells. Most of them can be synthesized.

Chemotherapy, treatment with chemotherapeutics.

Choriocarcinoma, a malignant tumour of the placenta.

Chromosomes, structures in the nucleus of the cell that can be stained.

A chromosome is essentially composed of the chromonema, a long twisted thread on which there are nodular structures, the chromomeres. The chief constituents of the chromomeres are deoxyribonucleic acids (DNA)-molecules or portions of these molecules. They carry the hereditary determinants, the genes (q.v.). The nuclei of the cells of each species have a definite number of chromosomes. The human body cell contains 46 chromosomes, in 23 pairs – i.e., two sets – one of which comes from the father and the other from the mother. In the mature germ cells, these sets divide during cell reproduction, each forming the basis for a new body cell. The chromosomes in each pair therefore resemble one another (autosomes). But exceptions are the sex chromosomes which are un-paired in the male. They are called X and Y. The female has no Y-chromosomes, but two X-chromosomes.

Cirrhosis, shrinkage and hardening of an organ, especially of the liver (liver cirrhosis).

Co-carcinogen, an additional cause of cancer or carcinogen.

Configuration, the form, shape or chemical structure of a molecule.

Cortex, rind, especially the adrenal cortex, which is part of the adrenal glands (glands which produce an internal secretion).

Corticosteroids, chemical compounds (steroids) which have the effect of the adrenal cortex hormones.

Cyst, a bladder-like, or saccular, closed space the contents of which are fluid or pulpy. Cysts are usually benign. If, however, they become very large and cause symptoms, they must be surgically removed. They can change into the form of cancer called a cystoma.

Cytology, the science of cells.

Cytoplasm, plasma – the fluid cell contents – surrounding the nucleus of the cell.

Cytostatics, drugs which inhibit cell growth.

Deoxyribonucleic acid, DNA, nucleic acid.

Dermatitis, inflammation of the skin.

Diagnosis, detection of disease.

Diathermy-knife, an electric knife, used in complex operations, such as the removal of a malignant tumour.

DNA, abbreviation for deoxyribonucleic acid. See nucleic acids.

Dysgenetic, dependent on disordered, defective hereditary disposition.

Dystrophy, a nutritional disturbance with symptoms of break-down in organs or parts of the body.

EFS,	enzyme-forming system.
Electrons,	very small particles with a negative charge. They are either bound to the atoms or occur free. Cathode rays, and also beta-rays, consist of free electrons. For the kinetic energy of electrons, see electron volt.
Electron volt,	abbreviation eV, the unit measurement of the energy of electrons in motion. $1 eV = 1.6 \times 10^{-12}$ erg, i.e. the energy which an electron gets by acceleration in passing through a potential of 1 volt. $1 MeV = 1{,}000{,}000 eV = 1.6 \times 10^{-6}$ erg.
Embryo,	the genus in its early stage of development; in man, up to about the beginning of the 3rd month of pregnancy. Embryology, the science of the development of the embryo.
Endogenous,	from within, arising internally.
Endocrine glands,	glands which produce internal secretions.
Endoscopy,	inspection of internal spaces in the body with a tube (endoscope) equipped with an illuminating device; see bronchoscopy, gastroscropy, mediastinoscopy, rectoscopy.
Entero-viruses,	a group of viruses which cause, among other diseases, infantile paralysis and diseases of the air passages.
Enzymes,	ferments, proteins formed in living cells which are able, as catalysts, to accelerate or slow down chemical reactions, but in so doing remain unaltered. Enzymes are particularly important to metabolism. Each enzyme has a specific task; thus saccharase splits only cane-sugar (saccharose), maltase splits only maltose. Because each enzyme has only a very limited task, there must necessarily be many of them.
Epidemiology,	the science of epidemics, of diseases that occur massively.
Epithelium,	the outermost cell-layer of the skin and of the mucosae; also the superficial covering of the hollow spaces inside the body.
Ergastoplasma,	areas in the plasma of the cell which especially tend to absorb basic stains. At times, threadlike or lamellar structures can be found with the light microscope in the ergastoplasm. Corresponding to the ergasto-

plasma are those areas in the cell plasma where structures possessed of granules which contain ribonucleic acid can be detected by the electron microscope.

Erysipelas, An inflammatory disease of the skin, caused by certain bacteria, traumatic or wound erysipelas.

Erythematodes, a disease of the skin, which appears chiefly on the face, and spreads in butterfly shapes. Red, sharply-outlined, foci sensitive to touch appear. The disease is presumably caused by auto-immunity. Women suffer from it more often than men.

Erythrocytes, the red blood corpuscles. They are smaller than the white blood corpuscles and are much more numerous in the blood. Normally there are 4.5–6 million erythrocytes in 1 cubic centimetre of blood. Human erythrocytes are round discs; they have no nuclei. They take their colour from the blood pigment haemoglobin, which itself is the agent by which they perform their most important task – to take up oxygen from the air in the lungs and transport it to the cells of the rest of the body. Erythrocytes are formed in the bone-marrow. If abnormalities in their size and form are detected in the blood picture, pathological changes in the body must be suspected.

Exogenous, arising, or acting, from the outside.

Ferments, see Enzymes.

Fibroblasts, cells in the connective tissue, predecessors of fibrocytes.

Fluorescence, luminescence shown by many substances when they are irradiated.

Gamma-globulins, proteins found in the blood plasma. They contain many antibodies and are therefore bearers of defences against infection. They can be obtained from the blood plasma and injected for the treatment of infectious diseases, such as chicken pox, measles, mumps and infantile paralysis, or for immunisation against them.

Gamma rays, rays of radioactive elements due to electromagnetic vibrations. Their wave length is even smaller than that of Röntgen rays, a fact which gives them a greater power of penetration. Especially used for the treatment of malignant tumours, they are artificially produced in the gammatron.

Gammatron, an apparatus for making gamma rays by means of a radioactive element, usually Cobalt 60, which sends out gamma rays as it disintegrates.

Gastritis, inflammation of the mucosa of the stomach.

Gastroscopy, inspection of the interior of the stomach with an endoscope introduced through the oesophagus.

Gene, the bearer of the hereditary predisposition. It occurs especially in the chromomeres – see Chromosomes. The genes consist of deoxyribonucleic acid (DNA) molecules, or portions of these.

Genesis, origin, development.

Genetics, the science of heredity, especially that of the the hereditary predisposition.

Genetic, concerning the hereditary predisposition or the history of development.

Genitals, the sexual organs.

Genotype, the hereditary structure, the whole of the hereditary predisposition. See phenotype.

Glioblastoma, a malignant tumour of the cerebrum. It grows rapidly and has a tendency to bleed.

Glioma, a general term for tumours of the supporting substance (neuroglia) of the nervous system and brain. Especially malignant is glioblastoma.

Gonadotropic, acting on the sexual glands.

Granulocytes, white blood cells formed in the bone marrow. Under the microscope, when they have been stained, fine granules can be seen in them. According to the nature of these granules, three kinds of granulocytes can be distinguished: neutrophils, eosinophils and basophils.

Haematopoiesis, the formation of the cellular constituents of the blood.

Haemoblatoses, malignant diseases of the blood-forming organs, such as leukaemia, reticulosarcoma, lymphogranulomatosis etc.

Haemoglobin, blood pigment, a protein, composed of the pigment haem and the protein globin. Red blood corpuscles are rich in haemoglobin and owe their colour to it. The pigment portion contains iron, which is necessary for combination with oxygen. It enables the red blood corpuscles to perform their most important function: to take up oxygen from the air in the lungs and carry it to the cells of the body. The estimation of the haemoglobin content forms part of the blood picture, q.v. The normal amount of 16 g. of haemoglobin in 100 cubic centimetres of blood in the male and 14.6 g. in the female is called 100 per cent. A haemoglobin content of between 80–100 per cent is normal. If it is lower than this, a pathological condition, for example, anaemia must be inferred.

Hepatoma, a tumour in the region of the liver.

Herpes, diseases of the skin and mucous membranes, in which there are disintegrating vesicles, for example, *herpes simplex* and *herpes zoster.* They are caused by viruses.

Histology, the science of tissues, especially of their structure and nature, and their individual constituents, the cells (cytology). Tissue is chiefly studied under the microscope. The commonest method of doing this is to make very fine sections of tissues, which are then stained, so that the individual kinds of tissues and their constituents are contrasted with one another. By this method diseased and tumorous tissues can also be assessed.

Histones, simple proteins, found in the nucleoproteins of the nuclei of cells and in the formed parts of the cell plasma.

Hodgkin's disease, lymphogranulomatosis, q.v.

Hormone treatment, treatment with hormones, as for example, the treatment of mammary cancer with male sexual hormones (the opposite hormones). If the hormone preparations cannot withstand the digestive juices, they must be injected under the skin or into the muscles. Hormones are also used in other diseases, for example, the treatment of diabetes with insulin.

Hormones, active substances characteristic of the organism. They are produced by the glands which make internal secretions and are discharged into the blood. They control the processes of metabolism, growth and development, and are of major importance to the organism. The pituitary gland occupies a key position among the glands of internal secretion. By its close connection with the midbrain it establishes the relationship between the formation of hormones and nervous system and its hormones regulate the activity of the other glands. The action of the individual hormones is very finely balanced; If one is absent, the action of the others is impaired; see hormone treatment.

Horror autotoxicus, "the fear of self-poisoning" according to Paul Ehrlich's axiom. He said that the body will not form antibodies against substances formed by itself – see autoantibodies.

Humoral, concerning the body fluids.

Hygiene, all measures that help in the prevention of disease and its spread.

Hyperplasia, the excessive increase and multiplication of certain cells and constituents of tissues.

Hyperthermia, overheating.

Hypertrophy, excessive growth of certain cells and tissues.

Hypophysis, the pituitary gland; see Hormones.

Hypoxia, lack of oxygen in the tissues.

Immunisation, protective inoculation, the artificial production of immunity. Active and passive immunisation are two different things. For active immunisation, vaccines are used. For passive immunisation, antisera are chosen (see blood serum).

Immunology, the science of immunity; immunological – concerning immunity.

Implantation, the implantation into the body of its own or foreign tissue. For example, cancer cells can be implanted for research purposes. One also speaks of implantation when metals, synthetic material etc. are put into the body to be enclosed there by healing. see Transplantation.

Induction, cause, especially in connection with the artificial production of tumours in experimental animals.

Infusion, introduction of large quantities of fluid under

the skin (subcutaneous infusion) or into the blood (intravenous infusion).

Initiation, introduction, beginning, first stage.

Internal secretion, the secretion of fluids (incretes) by certain glands directly into the blood. The incretes contain special active agents, the hormones. Among the glands that produce internal secretions (endocrine glands) are the hypophysis, the thyroid, parathyroid glands, adrenal glands, the pancreas, sex glands, the placenta, the thymus and the epiphysis; the hypophysis holds a key position. see Hormones.

Interferon, a protective substance formed in the cells in almost all virus infections, which inhibits the multiplication of viruses. The reaction between interferon and the virus varies according to the kind of virus. Interferon is chemically a protein.

intravenous, in or into the veins.

intracellular, inside the cells.

in vitro, in a test tube, research in artificial nutrient solutions – contrasted with *in vivo.*

in vivo, in the living creature: research on living organisms, in contrast to *in vitro.*

ionizing rays, rays which produce, as they penetrate matter, electrically charged particles, for example, the rays of radioactive substances, Röntgen rays.

Iso-antigens, tissue-specific antigens: antigens which are characteristic of a certain tissue or cell-type.

Isotope, modifications of chemical elements. They differ from their sources and from one another by their atomic weight. Otherwise they have the same nuclear charge, and therefore the same specific atomic number, and occupy the same position in the periodic system. There are stable and unstable isotopes. The latter are called radioactive isotopes or radionucleides.

Jensen Sarcoma, a very malignant sarcoma, of the rat, named after the Danish cancer investigator C. O. Jensen. It can be implanted into other animals.

Laser, light amplification by stimulated emission of radiation. An apparatus which amplifies and concentrates light so much that it acquires enormous energy. The rays emerging from a laser can bore through the hardest substances in a few seconds. Lasers are also used experimentally for the destruction of cancer cells.

Latent, remaining temporarily hidden, dormant. Present, without making an appearance.

Leukaemia, a disease of the blood-forming organs, nowadays classified as cancer, in which there is an enormous multiplication of the white blood cells (leucocytes). The two most important forms of the disease are myeloid (granulocytic) leukaemia and lymphatic (lymphocytic) leukaemia. Leukaemia may also be acute or chronic. In the myeloid form, granulocytes, and in the lymphatic form, lymphocytes, appear in increased numbers. Another feature of leukaemia is the appearance in the blood of immature white blood corpuscles. Because the number of blood platelets, which assist the coagulation of the blood, is decreased, leukaemia is accompanied by a tendency to haemorrhage; the spleen and lymph glands are enlarged, and other symptoms are anaemia, fever and pains in the joints and bones.

Leucopenia, the pathological reduction in the number of white blood corpuscles (leucocytes).

Leucocytes, the white blood corpuscles. They are bigger than the red blood corpuscles and much less numerous. For each white blood corpuscle there are about 600 red ones. In contrast to the red ones, the white blood corpuscles have a nucleus. Three kinds of white blood corpuscle are recognised according to their site of origin: the granulocytes (formed in the bone marrow), the lymphocytes (formed in the spleen and lymph glands) and the monocytes (the site of origin of which is disputed). The function of the leucocytes is to destroy bacteria that have penetrated into the body; they can also break down dead tissue and foreign bodies. The number of leucocytes in the blood is increased in suppurative diseases. It is pathologically increased in leukaemia, for example.

Lues, Syphilis.

Lymph, the tissue fluid. It is formed by the extravasation of fluid from the capillary blood vessels in the tissues. The system of lymphatic vessels conducts the lymph back to the blood circulation. The lymph glands, which belong to this system, act as filters which intercept bacteria, toxins, etc.; in so doing, they may become enlarged. The cells of malignant tumours are also filtered by the lymph glands, which in this way prevent the immediate flooding of the whole body with tumour cells.

Lymphogranulomatosis, Hodgkin's disease, a severe, tumour-like disease of the lymphatic tissues (lymph glands, spleen, liver, etc.) Symptoms are: enlargments of the lymph glands, especially those of the neck, pruritus, sweating, atypical fever, extreme emaciation and anaemia.

Lymphoid, lymph-like.

Lymphoma, a hypertrophy, proceding from the lymph glands.

Lymphosarcoma, a malignant tumour of the connective tissue.

Lymphocytes, white blood corpuscles formed in the spleen and in the lymph glands.

Lysis, dissolution.

Macromolecule, a giant molecule, see molecule.

Macrophages, cells which can ingest, feed on, and digest other cells. They may pass into the blood and take part in the battle against foreign elements that have got into the body (bacteria).

Malignoma, name for a malignant tumour.

Mamma, the female breast glands, which, with the fat and connective tissue around them, form the breasts.

Mammary cancer, breast cancer, cancer of the glands of the breast, malignant tumour of the breast glands – all show hardenings or nodules in the breast as their symptoms.

Mammography, a representation of the breast-glands by means of X-rays, often achieved with the aid of a contrast medium introduced into the glands of the breast. It is used to detect pathological changes in the breast – especially cancer.

Mediastinoscopy, inspection of the mediastinum, the middle part of the thoracic cavity, by the introduction into it of a tube provided with an illuminating device.

Medulloblastoma, a malignant tumour of the cerebellum. Medulla = the continuation of the spinal cord. A medulloblastoma grows rapidly. It occurs chiefly in children and young adults.

Melanoblastoma, a melanoma, q.v.

Melanoma, a tumour of the skin, mucosa of the eye, and occasionally of the membranes of the brain. It is a pigmented tumour usually malignant, containing large quantities of the pigment melanin, and it grows very rapidly.

Metabolism, all the processes which serve for the synthesis, reconstruction and decomposition of constituents of the body: respiration, digestion, assimilation, excretion and exchanges in the cells.

Metabolites, active agents; substances which are absolutely necessary for metabolism. Examples of them are nucleic acids, amino acids, hormones, enzymes and vitamins.

Metastasis, a secondary tumour; the detachment of tumour cells from the main or primary tumour. The cells are usually carried in the blood or lymph to distant parts of the body, where they settle and grow into secondary tumours.

meV, Mega (= million) electron volt.

Microbiology, the science of small forms of life.

Micron, one thousandth of a millimetre.

Microsomes, fine, granular structures in the cell plasma. They are the sites of protein synthesis.

Millimicron, a millionth part of a millimetre.

Mitochondria, thread-like or rod-shaped structures in the cell plasma. They are the vehicles of respiration and other metabolic processes.

Mitosis, the process of nuclear division.

Molecule, the smallest unitary particle of a chemical compound. A molecule consists of two or more atoms. The molecules of proteins may be composed of several million atoms and are therefore so large that they can be detected by the electron microscope (macromolecules).

Mongolism, an inborn form of feeble-mindedness caused by an anomaly in the chromosomes. When the chromosomes undergo division, the separation of one pair of chromosomes does not occur. The result is that, in fertilisation, an embryo is formed in which chromosome (autosome) No. 21 is trebled (trisomy) instead of doubled. The mongoloid person thus has one chromosome too many. Symptoms of the condition are a mongoloid appearance (slit-like eyes), saddle nose, malformation of the ear muscles, flabby muscles, joints that can be over-extended and (frequently) cardiac defects. Mongolism is often accompanied by leukaemia.

moribund, at the point of death.

Morphology, the science of the form and structure of the body and of its parts; morphological – relating to the form.

mutagenic, causing a mutation.

Mutation, a sudden change in the hereditary disposition, so that altered hereditary characteristics appear. The change affects the genes. It is possible to cause mutations artificially by means of ionising rays or chemical substances.

Myelocytes, early stages of granulocytes.

Mycoplasmata, PPLO, (Pleuro-pneumonia-like organisms), small polymorphic organisms. Their size is between that of bacteria and viruses. In contrast to viruses they have their own particular metabolism, and can be cultivated in certain cell-free nutrient fluids.

Myxo-viruses, a group of viruses which cause, among other diseases, influenza and mumps.

Necrosis, the death of tissues and organs.

Neutrons, elementary particles, in the nuclei of atoms, which have no electrical charge. They are set free in nuclear reactions; having marked pentrability they are used in the treatment of malignant tumours.

Nucleic acids, important constituents of the cell nucleus and of the formed parts of the cell plasma. They are compounds composed of a base (purine or pyrimidine) a pentose (ribose, deoxyribose) and phosphoric acid. Ribonucleic acid occurs in the cell nucleus and plasma, and deoxyribonucleic acid occurs in the chromatin of the cell nucleus, especially in the chromomeres of the chromosomes. Molecules or portions of molecules of deoxyribonucleic acid make up the genes.

Nucleoli, small bodies in the nucleus of the cell.

Nucleoproteids, see proteids.

Nucleotides, units of construction of the nucleic acids.

Oedema, dropsy; pathological accumulation of fluid in the tissue spaces.

Oncogenic, causing tumours.

Oncology, the science of tumours, particularly those which are malignant.

Oncolysis, the disintegration of a tumour.

Organotropic, related to or acting on a certain organ.

Oestrogens, originally only the name for the hormones which cause "heat" in female animals. Nowadays, however, many female sex hormones are called oestrogens. They not only affect the female sex organs, but also the skin, bone-marrow and many processes in the cells and tissues.

Ovarium, plural; ovaries. The ovary.

Papilloma, a benign or malignant tumour composed of connective tissue rich in blood vessels, with an epithelial covering.

pathogenic, causing disease.

Pathogenesis, the causation of disease.

Pathology, the science of diseases; pathological – diseased, abnormal.

Perfusion, administration of fluid to an organ or region of the body by means of an artificial circulation. During perfusion, the part of the body concerned is cut off from the general circulation.

Pernicious anaemia, one of the primary anaemias, which depends on the inability of the body to take in sufficient vitamin B_{12}. As a result of the lack of this vitamin, disturbance occurs in the maturation of the red blood corpuscles. They become abnormally large and rich in pigment, and there is a tendency to haemolysis. Other signs of the disease are a straw-coloured complexion and a smooth tongue; the patient feels weak, suffers from a burning tongue and paraesthesiae (itching, numbness) on the hands and feet.

Phages, bacteriophages.

Phagocytes, cells which can feed on and digest other cells. Among them are the macrophages and the microphages (see leucocytes.).

Phenotype, the outward manifestation determined by the hereditary disposition and the influences of the environment. See genotype.

Pharmacology, the science of drugs.

Physiology, the science of the life processes in the body.

Plasma, see blood plasma, cytoplasm (cell plasma).

Plasmagenes, genes present in the cell plasma, in contrast to the genes present in the cell nucleus.

Placenta, an organ which serves for metabolic exchanges between the mother and the foetus (unborn child). In addition, the placenta is an important gland producing an internal secretion.

Pleuropneumonia, simultaneous inflammation of the pleura and lungs.

Pneumonectomy, removal of a diseased lobe of the lung by operation.

Polio(myelitis), infectious infantile paralysis caused by viruses.

Polyoma virus, a virus which causes many kinds of malignant tumour in animals.

Polyps, tumour-like outgrowths of mucous membranes. They may develop in the nose, stomach, intestine, urinary bladder and uterus. They are benign, but sometimes cause trouble and need to be removed by operation. They may become cancerous, and must then be kept under observation.

polyvalent, acting in many ways, for example, against several causes of disease.

Portio, the part of the uterus which projects into the vagina.

PPLO, pleuro-pneumonia-like organisms, see mycoplasms.

precancerous, *precarcinomatous,* relating to the early stage of cancer or favourable to, or preparatory to, cancer. *Precanceroses,* are diseases which may lead to cancer, such as asbestosis, chronic gastric ulcer, chronic inflammation of the milk ducts or nipples, or of the breasts, also the scars of burns, white patches on the mucosa (leucoplakia), smoker's catarrh, X-ray and radium burns.

precarcinomatous, precancerous.

Promotion, the middle stage of development (of cancer).

Properdin, a protein component of the blood plasma – an endoglobulin of high molecular weight, belonging to the gamma globulins. Under certain conditions it can kill bacteria or neutralise viruses, or can dissolve pathologically altered red blood corpuscles.

Prophylaxis, the prevention of disease.

Prostate, the prostate gland, an organ which surrounds the first part of the male urethra.
Prostatic cancer, the malignant tumour of the prostate. Symptoms of it are retention of urine and rheumatism-like pains in the sacral region.

Protoamines, proteins of very simple structure, chiefly found in the sperms of fish.

Proteids, proteins in the wider sense. The protein molecules of the nucleoproteids are combined with nucleic acids. The nucleoproteids occur, among other places, in the cell-nucleus and in the formed constituents of the cell plasma.

Proteins, albuminous substances which, with few exceptions, contain only amino acids with other adsorbed or incorporated substances. Proteins may consist of hundreds of thousands of atoms. They are therefore large enough to be detected with the electron microscope (macromolecules). They are especially important for the life processes of the cell. The enzymes which are important for the metabolism of the cell are proteins in the wider sense – proteids.

Proteolytic, decomposing or digesting substances.

Protoplasm, the living contents of the cell.

r, unit of measurement for Röntgen and Gamma rays. The amount of rays which generates ions in 1 cubic centimetre of air at 0 degrees C. and an atmospheric pressure of 760 mm. of mercury, and which altogether carries an amount of electricity of one electrostatic unit of both signs.

Rad, the radiation dose absorbed. Unit of measurement of the dose of Röntgen and other ionising rays. 1 rad. corresponds to an absorbed energy of 100 erg per 1 g. of mass (tissue).

Radicals, very reactive atom groups, which can start a reaction, but are only rarely stable when they are uncombined.

Radioactive isotopes, the radionucleides.

Radioactivity, the property possessed by certain chemical elements of breaking down and sending out rays (alpha, beta and gamma rays). In this process they change into new elements. In addition to the natural radioactive elements, such as Uranium, Radium and Thorium, artifical radioactive elements are now possible, and radioactivity has become very important in medicine: irradiations, see Beta-rays, gamma-rays, radionucleides.

Radiology, the science of radiation, of rays (radioactive rays, Röntgen rays, etc.) and their use.

Radiomimetic substances, substances which act in a similar way to ionising rays and can, for example, cause mutations in germ cells.

Radionucleides, radioactive isotopes; modifications of chemical elements which emit ionising rays. They have become very important in the diagnosis and treatment of various diseases, particularly cancer. The ability of many malignant tumours to store up certain radionucleides has made it possible to detect the site of the tumour with the aid of a Geiger Counter. The radionucleides are injected into the blood, which carries them to the place where they are preferentially stored. For example, radiophosphorus helps in the diagnosis of tumours of the brain and of breast cancer. Radioiodine is used in the treatment of cancer of the thyroid.

Rectoscopy, inspection of the rectum with a tube (rectoscope) which has an illuminating device and a bellows for unfolding the mucosa of the gut. The rectoscope also has a device which makes it possible to remove mucosa for examination.

Regeneration, restoration, new formation, healing.

Remission, transient improvement of a disease.

Replication, also reduplication; the exact copying of a substance, a protein or a virus particle in the living cell.

Resistance, the inborn ability to resist an infection or a poison. The causes of resistance have not yet been explained in detail. Resistance must be distinguished from immunity.

Respiratory tract, the air passages: the nose and throat region, the larynx, air tubes, bronchi.

Reticulo-endothelial system a system of very active reticulum and endothelium cells. It can destroy foreign bodies (bacteria) and form and store up anti-bodies. The cells composing it occur especially in the bone-marrow, spleen, liver and lymph glands, and also in the blood and lymphatic vessels. It is also called the resorbent internal surface of the body. It is important in the cure of many diseases, especially chronic conditions.

Reticulo-sarcoma, a malignant tumour of the reticulum cells, usually in the lymph glands; these become enlarged, and later fever develops.

Reticuloses, a name for various growths of certain cells (reticulum cells, endothelial cells) in the bone marrow, the lymph glands, spleen, etc. Malignant tumours of these cells also belong to the reticuloses.

Retinoblastoma, a malignant tumour of the retina of the eye. It occurs in children and young adults and is rare.

Retotheliosarcoma, reticulosarcoma.

Ribonucleic acid, RNA, see nucleic acids.

Rickettsias, small forms of life, between bacteria and viruses. They multiply only in living cells and cannot be cultivated on artificial media or in artificial fluids. They are found in fleas, lice, mites and ticks and can be transmitted to man. They cause various kinds of spotted fever (typhus).

RNA, an abbreviation for ribonucleic acid; see nucleic acids.

Röntgen rays, very short-wave electromagnetic rays discovered by Röntgen in 1895. They arise when electrons strike against solid bodies. This process is produced in Röntgen tubes (electron tubes). Röntgen rays are distinguished by their high penetrability; they are used for irradiation of the body and its parts, and for making pictures of them (X-ray pictures). They have curative properties in skin diseases and tumours, but are especially used for the treatment of cancer.

Rous-sarcoma, a transmissible sarcoma of hens, caused by the Rous-sarcoma virus, named after the American virologist Peyton Rous (pronounced Raus).

Sarcoma, the malignant tumour of the connective and supporting tissues.

Secretes, the fluid formed and discharged by glands.

Secretion, the discharge of fluids (secretes) by glands, either to the exterior (skin, mucosa) or to the interior (blood); see internal secretion.

secondary, in the second place, following after, dependent upon.

Sedimentation rate, of the blood corpuscles; see blood sedimentation.

Sequences, sequels, series, portions (for example, of the constituents of a molecule).

Serum, see blood serum.

sessile, settled, sedentary.

Shope papilloma, see papilloma, a papilloma occurring in wild rabbits, which Shope was able to transmit to other wild rabbits.

Simian viruses, a group of viruses found in the kidney cells of monkeys (SV-viruses).

Smegna, a sebaceous secretion under the foreskin of the male penis, and in the female in the clitoris and between the lips of the vulva.

Soma, the body, *somatic,* relating to the body, corporeal; *soma cells,* body cells.

Sperm, semen, the seminal fluid, the secretion of the male genital glands in which the spermatozoa occur.

Spinalioma, a prickle cell cancer, a malignant tumour of the skin and mucosa, often at the transition between the skin and mucosa (lips, eyes, sex organs, scars, etc.), which at first looks like a wart. It tends to produce a running discharge and to suffer haemorrhages and ulceration.

Sputum, the mucus expectorated from the air passages by coughing. It may contain blood or pus. It is important in the diagnosis of diseases.

Steroids, chemical compounds, which include, among other substances, the sex hormones, the hormones of the adrenal cortex, the bile acids and vitamin D.

Stress, the burdening of the whole organism and of individual parts of it. The idea of stress was originated by Hans Selye (Montreal, Canada). The strain in the body due to infections, poisoning, injuries or psychological stimulation (stress-situation) causes increased secretion of the hormones of the adrenal cortex, as well as a compensating regulation of the anterior lobe of the hypophysis. The body seeks to adapt itself to the new situation. If it does not succeed, the "adaptation diseases" (skin diseases, allergies, rheumatism, blood diseases, etc) may appear.

Subcutaneous, under the skin.

Submicroscopic, not visible with the normal microscope.

Substrate, essential constituent, basis, substance, nutrient media.

Sulphonamides, chemotherapeutic drugs used against bacterial causes of disease. The basic constituent of them is sulphanilamide, which removes the p-amino-benzoic acid important for the metabolism of many bacteria. In this way the bacteria are killed, or so damaged that they can no longer multiply, they therefore succumb to the defensive substances of the body.

Supervolt treatment, the treatment of malignant tumours with very short-wave Röntgen rays or gamma rays.

Supersonics, sound waves which oscillate so rapidly that the human ear can no longer hear them. They are directed to the part of the body to be treated and can have therapeutic effects by means of warmth and massage.

Suspension, the floating of fine particles in a fluid.

Syncarcinogenesis, the co-operation of several carcinogenic factors which leads to the formation of a cancer.

Synthesize, to construct or make artificially by chemical methods.

Tobacco mosaic virus, the cause of leaf-spot disease of tobacco.

Therapy, the treatment of diseases.

Thoracotomy, opening the thorax in surgery. It is done either by cutting through the ribs or by entering the thorax between them (intercostal thoracotomy).

Thymus gland, a gland which presumably produces an internal secretion. It lies behind the upper part of the sternum, and consists of a cortex rich in lymphocytes and a medullary layer. When sexual maturity is reached it undergoes involution. There is a relationship between the thymus and growth.

Tissue, an association of cells of the same kind. The following kinds are distinguished: epithelial tissues, connective and supporting tissues, muscle and nervous tissues. The science of tissues is Histology q.v.

Tissue culture, the cultivation of cells and tissues in sterile nutrient media (*in vitro*). Such cultures permit observations to be made which would be impossible in the actual organism (*in vivo*). Tissue culture is a method for the observation of the metabolic and growth processes in cancerous tissue, and is also used for making virus vaccines. There are various methods of tissue culture.

toxic, poisonous.

Transfusion, transmission of a fluid, especially blood.

Transplantation, the transplantation of tissue. In autoplasty, the tissue transplanted comes from the same person; in homoplasty, from a different one. Heteroplasty, the transplantation of tissue from animals to man, has either only transient success or none at all. Complete success is attained only with autoplasty. Transplantation is used in experiments on animals; thus pieces of malignant tumours can be transplanted from one animal to another.

Tumour, an abnormal new formation of tissue, the cause of which is not directly ascertainable. There are benign and malignant tumours. The benign tumour does not exceed the proper tissue limits, whilst the malignant one pentrates into and destroys the nighbouring tissues and may form metastases (q.v.).

Ultraviolet rays, the invisible rays beyond the violet of the solar spectrum. They are short-wave rays whose wave lengths come close to those of the Röntgen rays. They can be artificially produced. They stimulate the formation of pigment in the skin and the formation of vitamin D (anti-rachitic). They are lethal to bacteria, and also have other curative factors. Overstrong irradiation of the skin may cause, among other things, injuries that cause or favour the development of skin cancer.

Uraemia, poisoning of the organism by substances which are normally excreted in the urine.

Urethane, ethyl carbamate, used for the treatment of chronic leukaemia; in experiments on animals it has a carcinogenic effect.

Urologist, a medical specialist in diseases of the urinary organs; see urology.

Urology, the science of the diseases of the urinary organs, kidneys, renal pelvis, ureters, urinary bladder, urethra.

Vaccine, originally smallpox vaccine derived from the cow (Latin: vacca). Plural, vaccines.

Virology, the science of viruses.

Virulence, attacking power.

Virus, minutes causes of disease in man, animals, plants and bacteria. Most viruses can be made visible by the electron microscope (and some by the light microscope). In the core of each virus is nucleic acid, which is the bearer of hereditary characters (see nucleic acids). This is surrounded by protein. In large viruses there are other substances, such as lipoids. Viruses have no metabolism of their own; they grow and multiply only in living cells which they ultimately destroy or make malignant. Most viruses can be cultivated in tissue culture or in chick embryos. Among virus diseases are influenza, infantile paralysis, measles, mumps, small pox, rabies and foot and mouth disease.

Vitamins, organic substances necessary to life, which the organism must obtain from its food. Vitamins are made by plants and by bacteria. The daily requirement of vitamins is small, but if they are lacking or the provision of them is defective, symptoms of diseases (avitaminosis, diseases due to lack of vitamins) appear. Among diseases due to lack of vitamins are scurvy, beri-beri and rickets. Many vitamins are constituents of enzymes.

Xeroderma pigmentosum, light shrivelled skin. A rare inherited disease depending on increased sensitivity of the skin to light and especially to ultraviolet irradiation. The disease begins in early childhood with reddenings of the skin which are transformed into spots of pigment. The skin shrivels. Deformities occur on the nose, mouth and eyelids; at a later stage there are wart-like structures which may become malignant.

INDEX OF PERSONS

SUBJECT INDEX